'In all th[...]
weight [...]
direct as you have. I sincerely wan[...]
f*cking fabulous. I feel that the rest of my 30s will be
more successful and emotionally/mentally/physically
healthy for finding you.' Elisa, USA

'I was miserable, overweight and had back
problems at 24 years old. Your account
has unlocked the simplicity of weight loss
for me. I have lost 15kg and have a healthy
BMI for the first time in my adult life. I
understand food. My back problems have
gone! Thank you for empowering me to
change my life.' Rosie, Australia

'I just wanted to say thank
you. I have been doing a
slimming club for over a
year and have such a bad
relationship with food
because of it. I already
see a difference in my
relationship with food and
that's thanks to you. Thanks
so much.' Victoria, UK

'Since following you
I've had the healthiest
relationship with food with
balance and sustainability
in my diet. I can't thank you
enough.' Ellys, UK

'I just want to say a huge thank you
because you clarify so much in this insane
jungle of dieting. As someone who still
feels lost and shaken by anything food-
related you are some kind of safe haven. I
am genuinely grateful for that.' Laurel, USA

'I developed such an unhealthy relationship with food,
believing I should just be living off ridiculous crash diets
to lose weight and wondering why it was never working.
I've lost weight after a couple of months already and can
still treat myself to naughty things. I feel more balanced
again, so thank you.' Harriet, UK

EAT WHAT YOU LIKE

& LOSE WEIGHT FOR LIFE

'If you want to lose weight then this book is for you. Graeme has managed to explain the true (and only) mechanism behind weight loss using easy-to-understand images. His recipes are not only nutritious and balanced, but delicious too: showing you how to lose weight in an enjoyable sustainable way for life.'

NICHOLA LUDLAM-RAINE
Registered Dietitian as seen on BBC, ITV & Channel 4

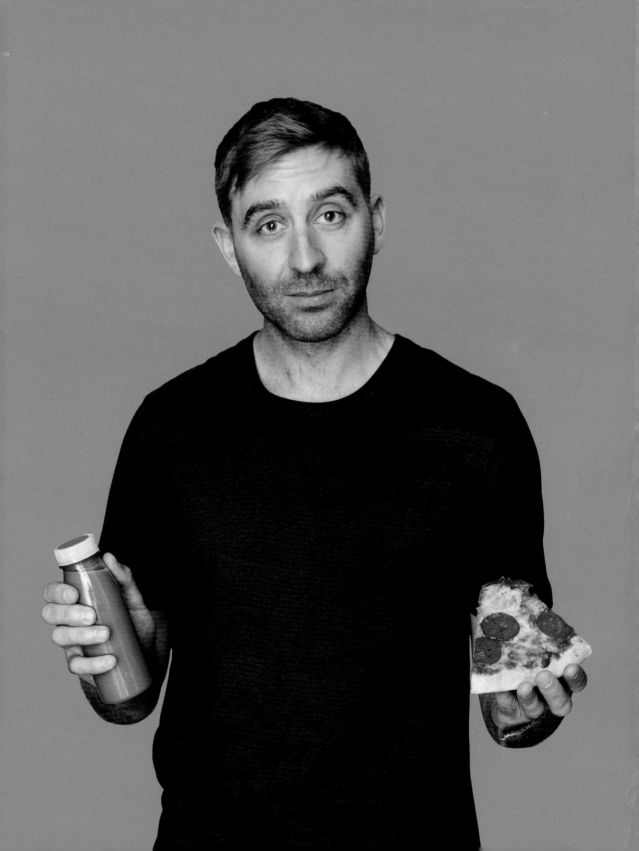

EAT WHAT YOU LIKE
& LOSE WEIGHT FOR LIFE

THE INFOGRAPHIC GUIDE TO THE ONLY DIET THAT WORKS

Graeme Tomlinson

EBURY
PRESS

CONTENTS

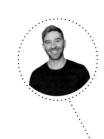

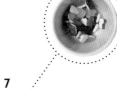

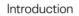

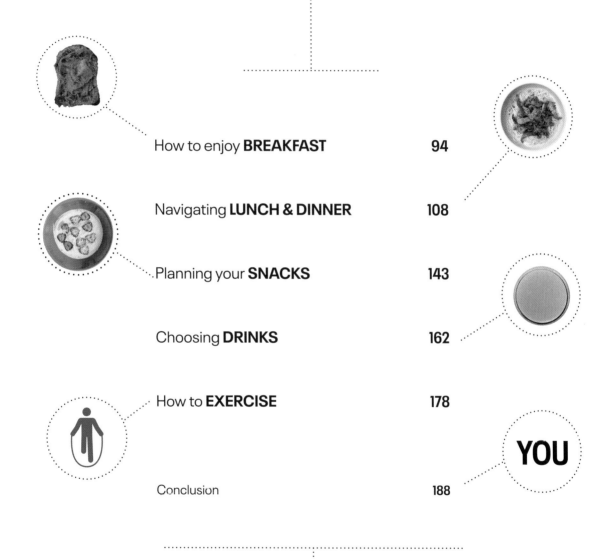

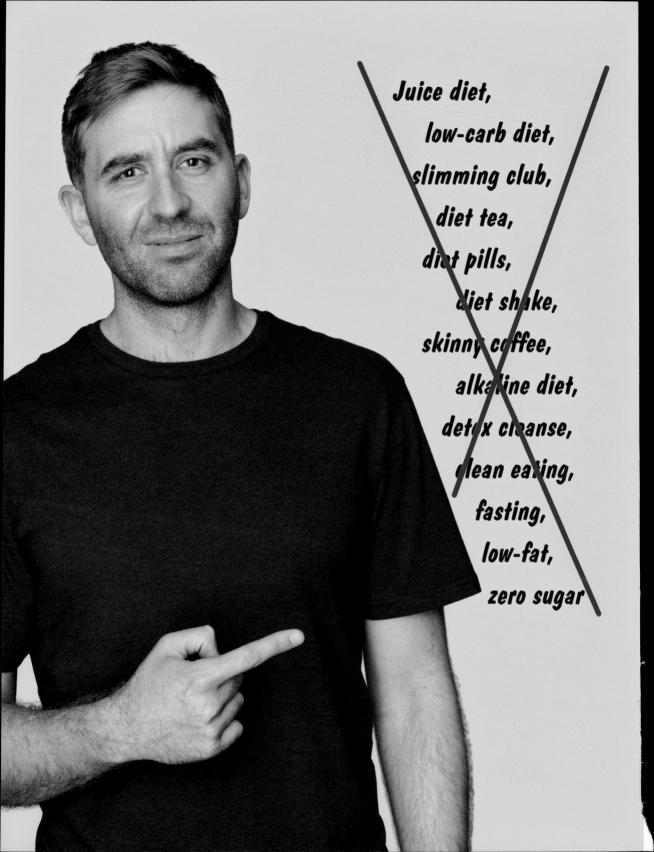

Juice diet,
low-carb diet,
slimming club,
diet tea,
diet pills,
diet shake,
skinny coffee,
alkaline diet,
detox cleanse,
clean eating,
fasting,
low-fat,
zero sugar

INTRODUCTION

What is the most effective way to lose weight and keep it off? There are so many diets available, each claiming that their method is best. How do you choose? Some say you should reduce carbs or restrict specific foods, others say you should fast for long periods of time or eat more frequently. Maybe a meal plan from a fitness celebrity is the answer? Or how about banning sugar from your diet?

The truth is: the only way to lose fat is to burn more calories than you consume.

For any fat-loss diet to work, it has to be based on the simple principle of what is known as **a caloric deficit.**

No prescriptive diet has been proven to make you lose weight unless it involves a state of overall caloric deficit, and all the 'weight-loss' diets and clubs out there ultimately offer alternative ways of achieving this.

Maybe this doesn't seem like such a bad idea. Following a prescribed diet makes life easier – there's no need for you to personally evaluate your food intake, you simply follow their rules, right?

No!

In my work as a personal trainer and nutrition coach, I see these complex and restrictive diets causing people to lose sight of the simple principles necessary for weight loss to occur. As anyone who has tried to stick to a prescribed diet knows, eliminating foods you enjoy or missing meals isn't easier than watching your portion sizes – and in any case, you still need to watch your portion size on any diet for it to work.

Diet Guilt

Your journey to lose weight should never begin because somebody else made you feel inadequate as you are. You should never feel external pressure to lose weight. Losing weight will only have a positive impact on your life if you recognize that doing so will improve the quality of your life. You have to have this self-motivation yourself.

What's more, many diets involve regimented recipe preparation, adding pressure to our increasingly busy days. Then you're asked out for a meal. You're offered a glass of wine or a slice of pizza, and sharing a good time with friends feels as important for your happiness as reaching your desired weight. You deviate. The next day, you feel like a failure. Now what's the point of continuing? You might as well abort this new eating regime because you can't stick to it.

Rigid diet schedules are as likely to lead to anxiety, guilt and discouragement as they are to weight loss, and with the volume of 'eat this, not that' rhetoric echoing across the media, deciding what to eat has become prohibitively complicated.

Most of us know that salad is nutritious. But what most of us don't know is that we can still eat things we love – chocolate, crisps, etc. – without feeling that we've failed, and still lose weight. This book will teach you how and why.

Exercise Fails

Too many of us are stuck in the rigid mentality that extreme, pulverizing exercise is essential if we want to burn fat. But, much like the restrictive and unnecessary diets that exist, this type of exercise is usually unsustainable. I will help you understand the basics and free you from the dreaded bootcamp mentality, because there are more enjoyable, sometimes surprising, but just as effective ways to exercise for fat loss. Much like eating food, if you don't enjoy what you're doing, you won't stick to it. So pick something you enjoy.

You Don't Need a New Diet

You already have a diet – what you eat every day. However, if your body composition isn't currently what you want it to be, you need to understand your daily diet a little better and make some adjustments.

The original definition of the word 'diet' is: 'The food and drink usually eaten or drunk by a person or group'. Now, 'diet' or 'dieting' most commonly refers to the attempt to alter body composition – usually for fat loss – by prescribed means. And as the world becomes more extreme, so do the diets. This simple deceptive noun, 'diet', has been transformed into an extreme, restrictive and unsustainable array of eating patterns and a guilt-invoking verb, 'dieting'. It's time to stop that.

Losing Weight and Enjoying Life

The aim of this book is to explain why you don't need to follow the likes of low carb, intermittent fasting, clean eating, slimming clubs, juicing and all the other restrictive dieting methods in order to achieve fat loss. It will show you a way to lose weight that's proven to be effective and doesn't ban any food types.

The only fat loss diet that works is the one that you can stick to consistently while enjoying your life. You just need to make a few small changes to ultimately get big results.

Using the simple principles in this book, you can take control of how you eat and manage your weight for the rest of your life, without cutting out any food groups.

There will be no temptation to return to unsustainable fad dieting trends after reading this book. All the information you need is presented in a series of powerful visuals to make sure that you understand exactly how to manage the food you eat, incorporate everything you enjoy and achieve your nutrition goals for the rest of your life. **No agenda. No gimmicks. Just facts.**

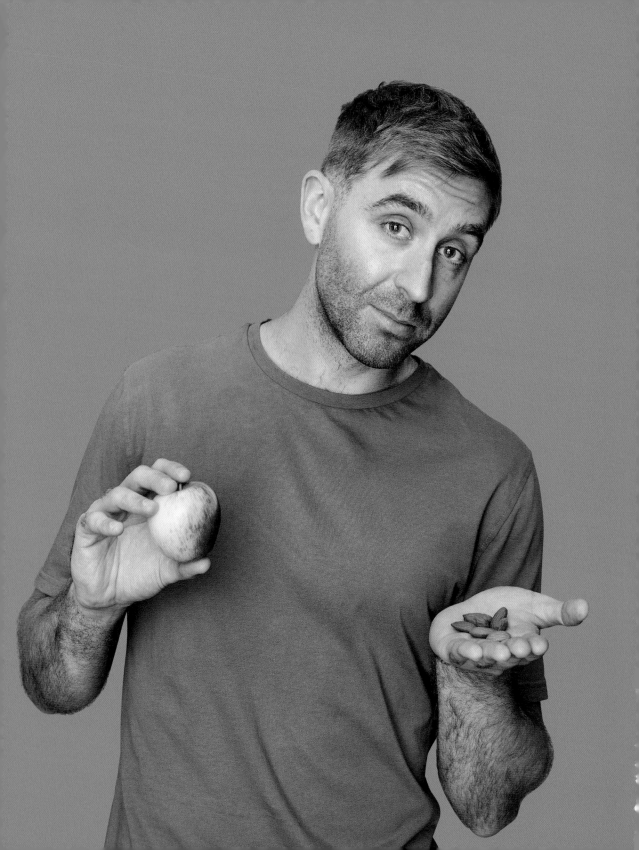

ABOUT ME

I started my Instagram feed in 2016 to post recipes for my followers, but by March 2018, having grown disillusioned with the unregulated nature of the fitness and diet industry, I started posting about the ironies, myths and pitfalls of dieting. My posts got people talking and distinguishing diet truths from diet fiction. The conversation continued, and by August 2019 more than half a million followers had joined in, including influencers and professionals, the national press and blogs worldwide. The more people who are able to arm themselves with information that can help them to better understand the basics of nutrition and improve their relationships with food, the happier I am.

My mission is to guide you through the maze of diet culture and food advertising, to provide you with an evidence-based resource and a practical perspective on food that you can use for the rest of your life to benefit your health. With each page of this book, you will silence the ingrained voice of the diet culture and replace it with a healthier, factual perspective on the food you eat.

Don't forget that food should be enjoyed, regardless of your fitness goal, so don't punish yourself with a dieting method you hate. The best way to lose weight is finding a diet that you can stick to consistently and enjoy. It is possible to get sustainable results and still eat chocolate, pizza or any other food you adore.

Many books tell us that their own rigid method is the only way to lose weight, but this book is different because I provide the information you need, back it up with science and deliver it with empathy and humour. The magic occurs by, crucially, allowing you to learn and become free to choose what you eat for yourself. This is how to bring about change.

For too long we have become slaves to misinformation and assumptions about nutrition, based on misleading dieting rhetoric. So we're going to start by looking at those diet myths and anecdotal theories about food and replace them with evidence-based information that will serve you better. Being aware of the basic principle required for fat loss will empower you to make informed decisions that will always support your goals.

Nutrition is a broad term. It encompasses a vast sphere of information and it means different things to different people. My aim is to find ways of presenting what is relevant in bite-size chunks, to change your mindset from paranoid, anxious, fearful and confused to optimistic, self-managing, empowered and informed.

A few notes
If you're used to cooking with cups and imperial measures, do not be put off that all the measures in this book are in grams. Grab yourself some inexpensive electric scales and select the gram measure. While you get to grips with calories, it is best to be accurate with your weight measures for ingredients and this is the simplest way to do that.

Where I use gram weights, as a rough guide:
1g = 0.035 ounces while 100g = ½ cup = 3.5 ounces.

Most of the nutritional information in the book is universal, with exception of some branded items which may have small or surprisingly large variations from one country to the next (e.g. a MacDonald's large fries = 510 kcal US and 444 kcal in UK; a Starbuck's chocolate brownie = 480 kcal US and 338 kcal UK, and a can of Sprite = 140 kcal US and 46 kcal UK). Branded products in this book share the UK calorie counts taken from their labels at the time of going to print. Always check the calories marked on the labels of products you are consuming.

Finally, information in this book has been sourced from the most recent meta analysis and systematic reviews – these are mass studies conducted on all existing research on any given question to ultimately give a reliable, objective answer. Too often people cite individual studies conducted in biased environments and believe the results to be definitive, not least the media.

HOW FAT LOSS WORKS – THE SIMPLE SCIENCE

THE CAUSE OF OBESITY IS SIMPLE

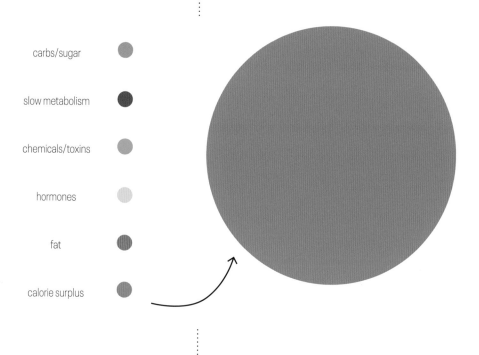

carbs/sugar

slow metabolism

chemicals/toxins

hormones

fat

calorie surplus

Despite what you hear in the media, or what friends may tell you, it is physiologically impossible to gain weight without a calorie surplus over time. Put simply, eating more calories than you use per day results in weight gain.

Many underlying things may contribute to weight gain. A calorie surplus may be the result of: choice, lack of nutritional understanding, belief in false information, disordered eating, food availability, a sedentary lifestyle, mental health or a combination of all. But a calorie surplus is always the resulting reason for weight gain.

THE TRUTH ABOUT
WHY WE ARE FAT

1990
28%* overweight (7% obese)

'fat is to blame'

* of total population

2005
36% overweight (10% obese)

'carbs are to blame'

2016
42% overweight (13% obese)

'sugar is to blame'

THE TRUTH

'NONE are to blame'

In 1975 only 23% of the world's population was classed as overweight (according to the World Health Organization), and only 4% was obese. In just 41 years that figure changed to 42% and 13% respectively, meaning that 1.9 billion adults are overweight and 650 million are obese. And 26% of western countries are classed as obese. In 1975 we ate fat, carbs and sugar. We also moved more. As each decade goes by, we move less. No one food type is to blame for these changing stats. Today we consume more calories than we burn, regardless of food/nutrient type. That's literally it.

Similar to the way trends in fashion shift over time, in the '90s the dieting industry demonized fat, because it is calorie dense. After the Millennium it was the turn of carbs, because reducing fat didn't stop obesity levels rising. And, more recently, it's been sugar, simply because it happens to be in those foods we eat in excess.

The truth is: none of these are to blame for the ongoing obesity epidemic. The reason for obesity is always the same: we eat more calories than we burn. The underlying cause for this caloric surplus may be the result of psychological, environmental or socioeconomic factors, but the science is always the same. We simply need to understand the food we eat a little better.

THE CRUCIAL ROLE OF ENERGY BALANCE

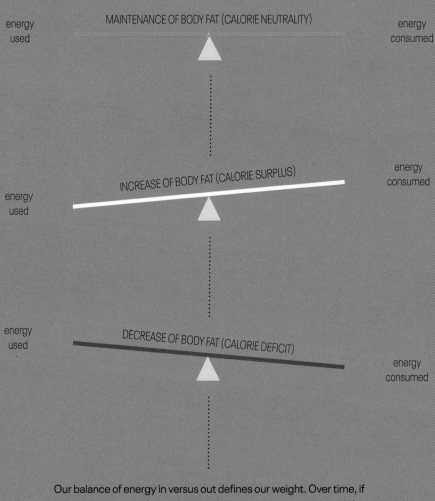

energy used

MAINTENANCE OF BODY FAT (CALORIE NEUTRALITY)

energy consumed

INCREASE OF BODY FAT (CALORIE SURPLUS)

energy consumed

energy used

DECREASE OF BODY FAT (CALORIE DEFICIT)

energy used

energy consumed

Our balance of energy in versus out defines our weight. Over time, if consuming more calories than you burn causes you to gain weight, then, naturally, consuming fewer calories than you burn will, over time, cause you to lose weight. This is referred to as a calorie deficit – the only physiological way a human being can lose weight.

THE CALORIE DEFICIT

A calorie is simply a unit of energy. When we consume calories our body stores them as energy to use. If we eat more calories than we use, we gain weight, but if we eat fewer calories than we use, we lose weight. It really is just that.

There are many expensive methods specially designed to lose fat, such as personal training sessions or choosing a diet where special ingredients are required, but none of them will work without a calorie deficit.

In simple terms, though 100 calories of carrots are more nutritious than 100 calories of chocolate, both store the same amount of energy.

DO YOU NEED TO FOLLOW A PRESCRIBED DIET?

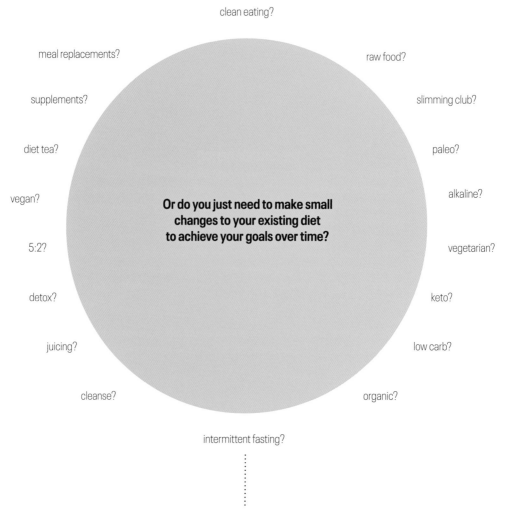

clean eating?

meal replacements?

raw food?

supplements?

slimming club?

diet tea?

paleo?

vegan?

alkaline?

Or do you just need to make small changes to your existing diet to achieve your goals over time?

5:2?

vegetarian?

detox?

keto?

juicing?

low carb?

cleanse?

organic?

intermittent fasting?

Unless you have a specific medical condition that requires the omission of certain foods or food groups, there is no good reason why you need to rip up your current diet and adopt a completely different diet to lose weight. There is only one principle that you need to focus on to lose weight and here we'll discuss its simple science.

FAT LOSS & FAT GAIN SIMPLIFIED

FAT LOSS

FAT GAIN

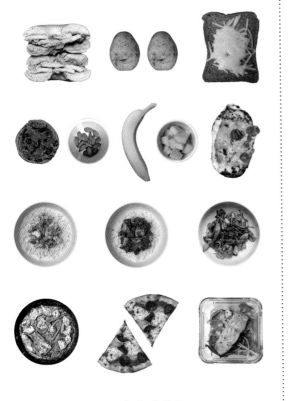

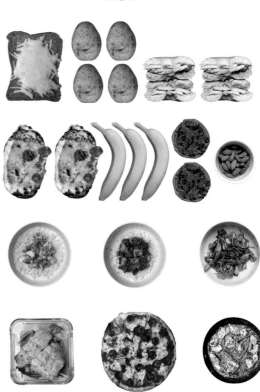

calorie deficit

eat fewer calories and move more

calorie surplus

eat more calories and move less

Despite the multi-billion-pound dieting industry, this graphic illustrates how simple the process of losing fat or gaining fat is.

HOW YOU CONSUME/BURN CALORIES

FOR MAINTAINING WEIGHT

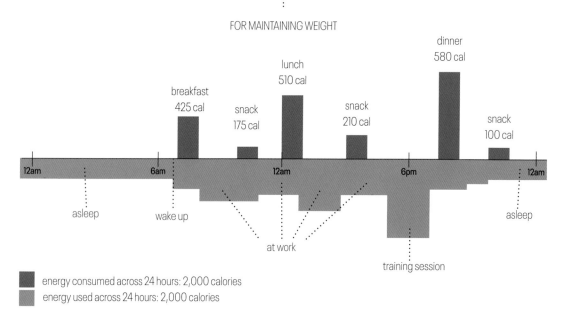

dinner
580 cal

lunch
510 cal

breakfast
425 cal

snack
175 cal

snack
210 cal

snack
100 cal

12am   6am   12am   6pm   12am

asleep

wake up

at work

training session

asleep

■ energy consumed across 24 hours: 2,000 calories
■ energy used across 24 hours: 2,000 calories

FOR GAINING WEIGHT

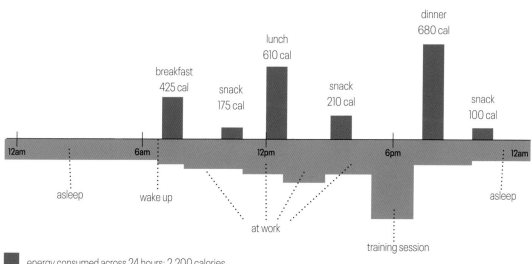

dinner
680 cal

lunch
610 cal

breakfast
425 cal

snack
175 cal

snack
210 cal

snack
100 cal

12am   6am   12pm   6pm   12am

asleep

wake up

at work

training session

asleep

■ energy consumed across 24 hours: 2,200 calories
■ energy used across 24 hours: 1,800 calories

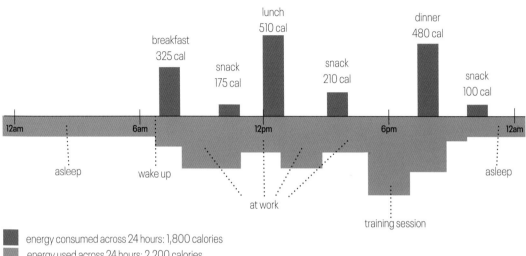

FOR LOSING WEIGHT

breakfast
325 cal

lunch
510 cal

snack
175 cal

snack
210 cal

dinner
480 cal

snack
100 cal

12am   6am   12pm   6pm   12am

asleep   wake up   at work   training session   asleep

■ energy consumed across 24 hours: 1,800 calories
■ energy used across 24 hours: 2,200 calories

These daily calorie targets are purely an example; yours will be unique to you. In terms of calories out, the graphics show that we burn the fewest calories when resting, moderate amounts when active during the day and the most in a short window of intense exercise. We consume calories from various meals and snacks throughout the day. The key is to understand your daily and weekly calorie needs to achieve your calorie deficit for fat loss. (See 'How to plan your calorie deficit', page 34.)

WHY CAN'T YOU LOSE WEIGHT?

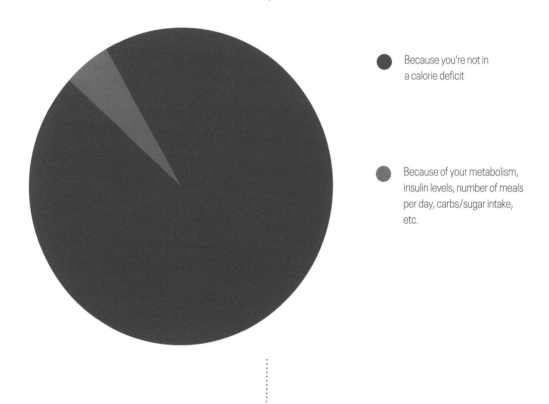

Because you're not in a calorie deficit

Because of your metabolism, insulin levels, number of meals per day, carbs/sugar intake, etc.

The simple answer to this question is that you are simply not in a calorie deficit. You may be underestimating or miscalculating the total calories you consume, or your target number of daily calories isn't actually supporting a calorie deficit. You may have also reduced the amount of energy you use each day, altering the energy balance out of a state of deficit. There is always a logical explanation. There are no mysterious fat-loss prevention demons – it is entirely scientific and can be explained every time.

UNDERSTANDING MACRONUTRIENTS

WHAT ARE MACRONUTRIENTS?

PROTEIN	CARBS	FAT
4 calories per gram	**4 calories per gram**	**9 calories per gram**

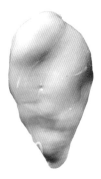

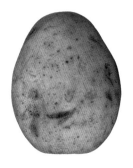

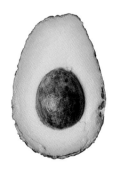

meat, poultry, whey, fish, seafood, dairy, eggs, pulses

fruit, vegetables, pulses, grains, sugar

avocado, nuts, oils, seeds, dairy, eggs

* alcohol contains 7 calories per gram

All of the calories that we consume are made up of varying amounts of different macronutrients. These are protein, carbohydrates, dietary fats and, to a lesser extent, alcohol.

Many of us get too caught up with macros. But macronutrients are essentially just different sources of energy that should all be included in a balanced diet.

Proteins, carbs and fats all give you energy. There are:

4 calories in every gram of protein
4 calories in every gram of carbohydrate
9 calories in every gram of fat
7 calories in every gram (or ml) of alcohol

People often get hung up about tracking macros instead of calories, but by tracking macros you are essentially tracking calories anyway.

UNDERSTANDING CALORIES, MACROS AND MICROS

CALORIES   CALORIES ARE DERIVED FROM MACRONUTRIENTS

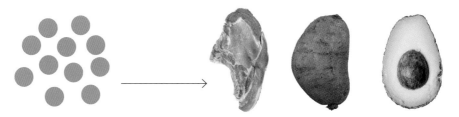

= units of energy   = proteins, carbs & fat

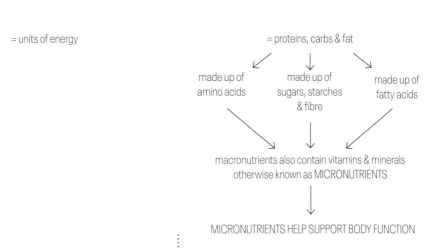

made up of   made up of   made up of
amino acids   sugars, starches   fatty acids
                    & fibre

macronutrients also contain vitamins & minerals
otherwise known as MICRONUTRIENTS

MICRONUTRIENTS HELP SUPPORT BODY FUNCTION

Calories are units of measurement found in food. Micronutrients are chemical elements within food that are required for the development of living organisms – and people say chemicals are bad. Micronutrients present themselves as vitamins and minerals within macronutrients. We consume calories, to give us energy, in the form of macronutrients. Calories directly influence how much body fat we have. Micronutrients don't contain calories and don't influence how much body fat we have , but do influence our function health.

BODY FUNCTION VS BODY FAT

DETERMINES
BODY FUNCTION

DETERMINES
BODY FAT

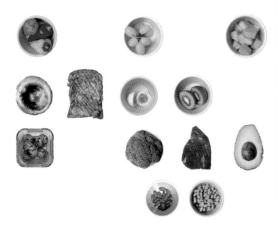

food that contains micronutrients

relies on food type

calories from all food

regardless of food type

This appears to be the greatest misunderstanding in nutrition history – and it doesn't help that 'nutrition gurus' often confuse foods that help your body function with foods that help you lose weight when talking about a healthy diet.

Micronutrients need to be present in your diet to help your body function – they contribute to healthy skin, strong bones and a good digestive system, for example. But they don't automatically reduce body fat. Only a calorie deficit can do that.

UNDERSTANDING PROTEIN

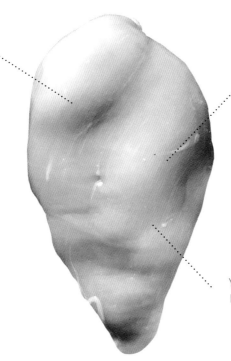

We digest protein more slowly than other macronutrients, which is why eating protein makes us feel fuller. It also supports the repair of our tissues and organs.

The human body burns more calories digesting protein (from the thermic effect of food, or TEF, see page 182) than it does other macronutrients (carbs and fat). Digesting protein burns 20-35% of the calories in it. So for 300 calories of pure protein consumed, around 60-105 calories are burned just through digesting it. Therefore eating protein increases your energy expenditure and also your calorie deficit.

Years of research show that a daily diet high in protein supports fat loss for the above reasons.

Whether you are male or female, I recommend you aim to consume 1–2g of protein per kilo of body weight per day to maintain muscle mass and keep you feeling full. If you train several times per week, you might need up to 2g per kilo of body weight.

For example, a female weighing 75kg (11st 8lb) can aim for 75–150g of protein per day. A male weighing 105kg (16st 5lb) can aim for 105–210g of protein per day.

UNDERSTANDING CARBS

Carbs give us energy to exercise and help our brain function.

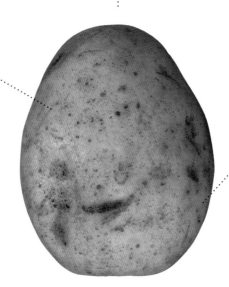

Digesting carbs burns 5-15% so for 300 calories of pure carbs consumed, around 15-45 calories are burned just through digesting it.

Ideally, carbohydrate intake should be based on high-fibre foods because fibre helps keep the body fuller for longer and also benefits gut health.

Wholefood carbohydrates, such as fruit, vegetables and pulses, also contain micronutrients, which support body function. Refined carbohydrates, such as bread and sweets, may not fill you up as much and usually contain fewer micronutrients and fibre, but of course you can still eat them.

Despite the demonization of refined carbs over the years, when it comes to fat loss, as with any food group, the key is that you appreciate the calorie value of any carbohydrate-rich food, not just its carbohydrate or sugar value.

UNDERSTANDING FAT

Important nutrients are present in sources of wholefood fat, such as avocados, nuts, seeds and oily fish. Other fats, such as butter, coconut oil and animal fats, contain fewer nutrients but are delicious.

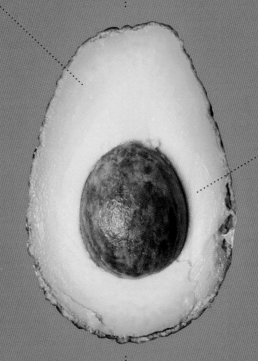

As with carbs, digesting fats burns 5-15% so for 300 calories of pure fat consumed, around 15-45 calories are burned through digesting it.

Fat is the most calorie-dense macronutrient, but that does not mean it is the enemy. If fat loss is your goal, you need to appreciate that all fats, including wholefood ones, come at a high caloric cost.

MACROS IN FOODS

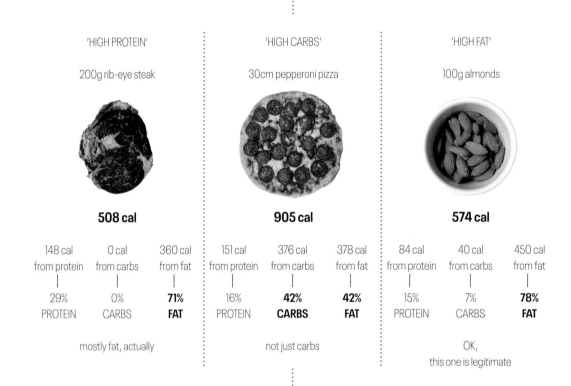

'HIGH PROTEIN'	'HIGH CARBS'	'HIGH FAT'
200g rib-eye steak	30cm pepperoni pizza	100g almonds

508 cal			**905 cal**			**574 cal**		
148 cal from protein	0 cal from carbs	360 cal from fat	151 cal from protein	376 cal from carbs	378 cal from fat	84 cal from protein	40 cal from carbs	450 cal from fat
29% PROTEIN	0% CARBS	**71% FAT**	16% PROTEIN	**42% CARBS**	**42% FAT**	15% PROTEIN	7% CARBS	**78% FAT**
mostly fat, actually			not just carbs			OK, this one is legitimate		

We often forget that individual foods labelled as 'high' in one macronutrient actually contain two or three macronutrients. Most food we consume contains all three macronutrients, so knowing the overall calorie value of a particular food is the most crucial step to losing weight, not macros. For example, a 200g rib-eye steak is often labelled 'high-protein', but out of 508 calories, only 148 are derived from protein; the remaining 360 are derived from fat. The rib-eye is high in protein compared with the other foods above (it contains 29% protein), but it's also high in fat (71% fat).

ALCOHOL

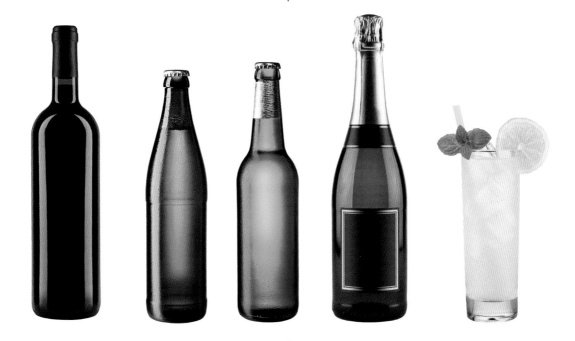

Although pure alcohol is, technically, a macronutrient, it offers little nutritional value and is fairly calorie dense (7 calories/g). All on top of the calories derived from alcohol itself. And while alcoholic drinks are not entirely made up from alcohol (otherwise we would die), the additional ingredients and mixers also contain calories. You can appreciate alcohol, if you like, but also appreciate its caloric cost.

FIBRE

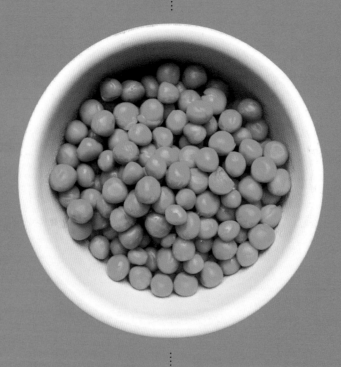

Dietary fibre is the parts of plants that cannot be broken down by enzymes in our digestive systems. Although fibre is a carbohydrate, it passes through the gut and is not, therefore, considered a macronutrient because it is not an energy source. We should eat high-fibre foods because they fill us up for longer, which helps prevent us from overeating. An added benefit of fibre is its role in supporting our gut health by absorbing water and keeping our bowel movements regular.

A BALANCED PLATE

salmon

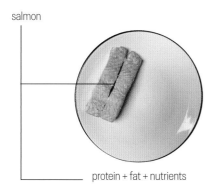

protein + fat + nutrients

pasta

vegetables

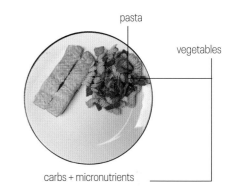

carbs + micronutrients

sweet chilli marinade (homemade)

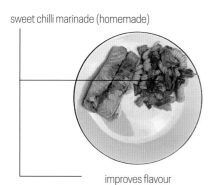

improves flavour

your twist

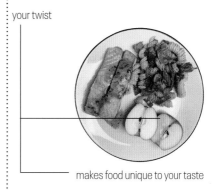

makes food unique to your taste

The above is a simple example of a balanced plate of food including protein, carbs, fats, micronutrients, flavour and an individual twist.

It is a good idea to ensure most of your main meals are balanced in all three macronutrients and include an abundance of micronutrients. A regular supply of all these things is needed to optimize a diet that supports any weight-related goal and your functional health. When building a balanced meal, first work out if it achieves your calorie and protein targets, then build the rest.

HOW TO PLAN YOUR CALORIE DEFICIT

HOW TO PLAN
YOUR CALORIE DEFICIT

A calorie deficit sounds simple; all you have to do is consume fewer calories than you use and you will lose fat. But people fail. This isn't because a calorie deficit doesn't work (it always works), it's just that the method didn't work. In truth, the most important question you should ask yourself when you begin planning your calorie deficit is: 'Can I adhere to this lifestyle for months and years and enjoy it?' If the answer is no then you need to find an alternative method. This chapter will show you how to sustain a calorie deficit, making small changes over time, which can lead to big changes in body weight with minimal upheaval.

Given that a calorie deficit is the only way to lose weight, it makes sense to understand the number of calories we consume to align the principle (calorie deficit) with your food behaviour (calories consumed).

A number of websites offer free calculators into which you can type information to obtain a daily calorie target for weight loss. The most popular formulas used by professionals include the Mifflin St. Joer, Harris Benedict and the TDEE method. The last of these simply calculates the total calories you use per day and produces a figure lower than this to ensure you consume fewer calories than you use. Check out my calculator (fitnesschef.uk) where you can quickly work out your daily and weekly calorie and protein requirements for weight loss.

WHY TRACKING CALORIES IS LIKE SAVING MONEY

YOU DO THIS...

SO WHY NOT THIS?

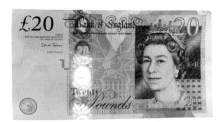

You
'Nibbles
don't count'
Reality
400 cal

You
'Fruit is
very healthy'
Reality
100 cal

You
'LOL, these don't
have calories'
Reality
250 cal

You
'Sh*t this must have
like 5,000 cal'
Reality
508 cal

You
'Need to eat
healthily after
that burger'
Reality
900 cal

You
'This is literally
no food at all'
Reality
50 cal

If you don't have enough money,
you don't go on holiday.

If you don't know how many calories you consume,
you don't know if you are losing fat.

The concept of counting your money in order to save enough to
go on holiday is very similar to counting the number of calories you
consume to ensure fat loss is achieved. Applying practical logic is
not obsessive – it's smart.

WHY YOU
SHOULD NOT CRASH DIET

7.30am breakfast

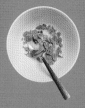

'Poverty bowl of fruit and fibre with skimmed milk
because I've been bad'
160 cal

12pm lunch

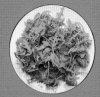

'The baked potato looks good, but I must have
this sad bowl of nettles instead'
160 cal

7pm dinner

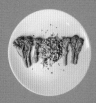

'I'm ravenous, but alas... some dry grains,
shrapnel and broccoli'
145 cal

7.10–10.30pm

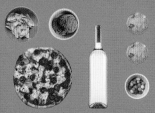

'I do not recall the past 2½ hours'
4,820 cal

We are an intelligent species. We require a calorie deficit for fat loss,
so logic tells us that in order to expedite fat loss as fast as possible,
we should eat as little as possible. But our intelligence also tells us
this is miserable. Naturally, this leads to an episode of binge-eating.

The irony is that our desperation for fast results increases our
likelihood of failure over time. To be intelligent about losing fat, we
must realize that success is entirely dependent on adherence. Only
then can you alter your approach from yo-yo dieter to happy eater
and from volatile weight swings to smooth progress, even if it is a
little slower.

HOW TO CALCULATE
A SUSTAINABLE CALORIE DEFICIT

Calories required to maintain
current weight (overweight)

3,500 cal

Deduct 15% from 3,500 cal
to create calorie target

2,975 cal

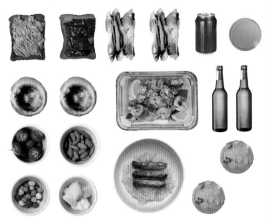

a few
months
later

New maintenance: 2,530 cal:
deduct 15% to create calorie deficit target

2,150 cal

New maintenance: 2,150 cal:
deduct 15% to create calorie deficit target

1,830 cal

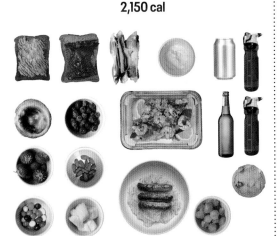
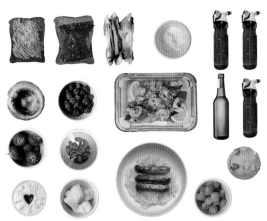

Along with understanding how many calories you need to achieve fat loss, you need to be able to ADHERE to and sustain it for it to work. If the calorie deficit is too aggressive, the chances of sustaining adherence reduces. A 15–20 per cent deficit from maintenance calories is advisable. Any lower and adherence becomes more difficult; any higher and the rate of progress may be frustratingly slow.

Though calculators (including mine) will work out a calorie deficit for you at the press of a button, it is useful to know how it is worked out. Age, gender, weight, height and activity level are assessed to produce a calorie requirement to maintain current weight, then a percentage is deducted to create a calorie deficit.

For example, if your total daily energy expenditure is 3,500 calories to maintain your current weight, to achieve a 15 per cent deficit, your new daily calorie target for fat loss would be 2,975 calories. Bear in mind that as you lose weight over weeks and months, you will have to keep recalculating your daily calorie target to keep losing fat. The leaner you become, the harder it is to lose fat at the same rate.

What about the macronutrient split? This is also worked out automatically for you by many calculators, including mine. The amount of protein you require (see page 27) will depend on your preference. You may feel full on 1g of protein per kg of bodyweight, or prefer up to 2g per kg of bodyweight. The remaining calories made up from carbs and fats can be consumed in whatever ratio you choose. The most recent meta-analysis suggests that low-carb or low-fat diets make no difference to the rate of fat loss when calories and protein are equated. So you can tell the tiresome low-carb enthusiasts to piss off. Do what you prefer.

You can log calories consumed using one of the many calorie-tracking apps available. But one negative most have in common is that they allow you to select rapid weight loss when you sign up. Ignore what they prescribe and simply use them to log the calorie target I give you using my calculator at fitnesschef.uk.

a few
months
later

New maintenance: 2,975 cal:
deduct 15% to create calorie deficit target

2,530 cal

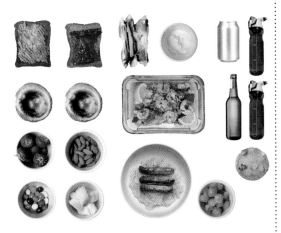

a few
months
later

1,830 cal

WHEN CONTENT, MAINTAIN
AWARENESS OF ENERGY
REQUIREMENTS RELATIVE
TO ENERGY USED

WHY TRACKING CALORIES WEEKLY COULD BE BETTER THAN DAILY

Most people track their calories daily. There is nothing wrong with that as such, but if you were to considerably exceed your daily calories and return to your calorie target the following day, it could be problematic because it is the average number of calories consumed over days, weeks and months that is important.

If your calorie target for fat loss is 2,000 calories per day, changing this to a target of 14,000 per week will give you the freedom to enjoy social occasions more, knowing that you will need to adjust your calories over the other days to ensure that your overall weekly target for fat loss can still be achieved.

daily target: 2,000 cal (14,000 per week)

weekly target: 14,000 cal

MONDAY   2,000 cal

2,000 cal

    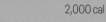

TUESDAY   2,000 cal

2,000 cal

WEDNESDAY   2,000 cal

2,000 cal

THURSDAY   **3,500 cal**

 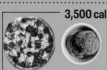

3,500 cal

 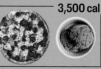

FRIDAY   2,000 cal

1,500 cal

SATURDAY   2,000 cal

1,500 cal

SUNDAY   2,000 cal

 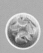 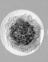

1,500 cal

  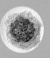

total consumed: 15,500 cal

exceeded target on Thursday, back on track the following
day, but the overall calorie deficit (14,000 per week) has not
been achieved.

total consumed: 14,000 cal

exceeded daily target on Thursday, but adjustments made over
the next three days to fit the weekly calore total. Success!
More flexibility = more adherence.

THE PROBLEM
WITH MEAL PLANS

A calculated meal plan provided by a fitness professional appears at first sight to be the platinum level of nutrition service. Recipes are tailored to your likes, dislikes, allergies and energy needs. But there is a problem with this system.

The graphic here illustrates what happens when you deviate from the plan – which is extremely likely if you have a social life. What occurs in this off-plan stage is unaccounted for. In your mind, it is the meal plan that achieves your goal, so if you fail at the meal plan you feel you have failed entirely. But these feelings of failure come from your inability to understand portion sizes, or to be flexible and know how to adjust your diet – because it's all been done for you.

What if Tuesday comes and you don't want the chicken and rice shown on your meal plan? What if you actually want something else? What happens at the end of the meal plan? Being empowered to make your own decisions and devise your own meal plan, based on your own knowledge, will be more enjoyable and more effective.

Following a set meal plan

MONDAY

TUESDAY

WEDNESDAY

THURSDAY

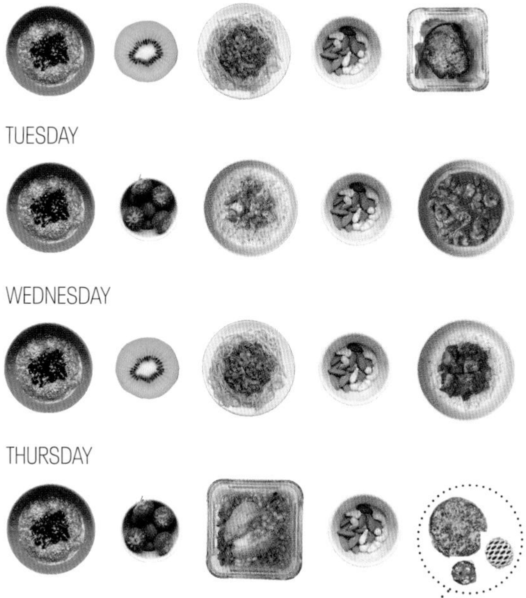

FRIDAY

Phoebe's birthday dinner (1,200 cal, off plan): 'I've ruined it all so I may as well give up.'

SATURDAY

WTF DO I DO NOW?

I ruined it all so I may as well give up

SUNDAY

clueless about energy balance and flexibility

Being flexible & accountable

MONDAY

TUESDAY

WEDNESDAY

THURSDAY

FRIDAY

SATURDAY

SUNDAY

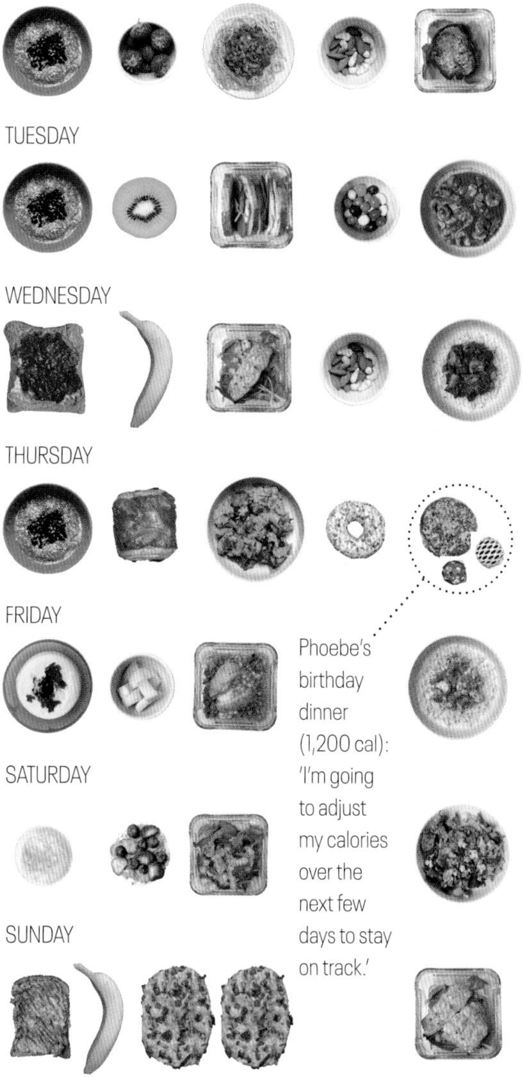

Phoebe's birthday dinner (1,200 cal): 'I'm going to adjust my calories over the next few days to stay on track.'

saved 600 calories from 3 days without afternoon snacks to stay on track

BEWARE
THE WEEKEND FAIL

MONDAY-FRIDAY

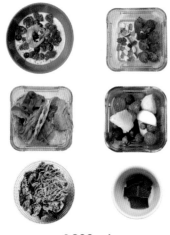

SATURDAY-SUNDAY

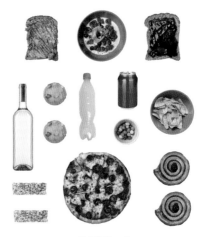

1,800 cal
per day

4,560 cal
per day

Individual's weekly calorie target: 12,600 calories, compared with
individual's actual weekly calorie intake: 18,120 calories.
A calorie deficit is not just for week days.

You may think that if you adhere to your fat-loss target 'most of the time' you will succeed, but you won't. Let's say your calorie deficit target is 1,800 calories per day (12,600 calories per week). If you consume 1,800 calories from Monday to Friday, but 'let your hair down' at the weekend, the implications of your weekend eating depend on the number of extra calories consumed. In this example, 4,560 calories are consumed on Saturday and Sunday, taking the total weekly calories to 18,120. This means that the overall weekly calorie target of 12,600 calories has been exceeded by 5,520 calories! If you want to let your hair down, do it, but make sure you stay within your calorie target for the week otherwise you will not lose weight.

WHY 'EYEBALLING' CALORIES IS HARD

PROBABLY MEASURED

PROBABLY UNMEASURED

90g avocado on toast

265 cal

30g peanut butter on toast

275 cal

180g avocado on toast

435 cal
(looks the same)

75g peanut butter on toast

545 cal
(looks the same)

30g cheese on toast

220 cal

30g choc & hazelnut
spread on toast

252 cal

75g cheese on toast

408 cal
(looks the same)

75g choc & hazelnut
spread on toast

500 cal
(looks the same)

Estimating calories by eyeballing food is only effective for those
trained and experienced in understanding the calorie density of
foods. Even if a serving of food looks the same, calorie values can
be very different. To determine accurate consumption, instead of
using your eyes, it's always best to read the labels and use scales to
track the calories you consume more accurately.

SAME FOOD, DIFFERENT CALORIES

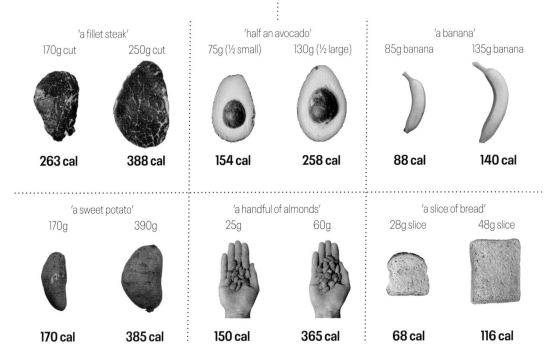

'a fillet steak'		'half an avocado'		'a banana'	
170g cut	250g cut	75g (½ small)	130g (½ large)	85g banana	135g banana
263 cal	**388 cal**	**154 cal**	**258 cal**	**88 cal**	**140 cal**

'a sweet potato'		'a handful of almonds'		'a slice of bread'	
170g	390g	25g	60g	28g slice	48g slice
170 cal	**385 cal**	**150 cal**	**365 cal**	**68 cal**	**116 cal**

Food items vary in size. Weighing some of these goods may be useful if weight loss/gain is the goal.

This image highlights that perceived 'standardized' measures of items of food, such as handfuls, halves and slices, may contain very different calorie values depending on the size.

If you track your nutritional intake on a calorie-counting app, you may believe that half an avocado is a generic measurement for all avocados. But any item of wholefood can greatly vary in size, thus altering its calorie value. If you ate the above items in one day without weighing them, you could consume 893 calories or 1,652 calories without registering the big difference.

'I DON'T KNOW WHAT
TO EAT FOR FAT LOSS'

what you currently eat

what you need to eat for fat loss

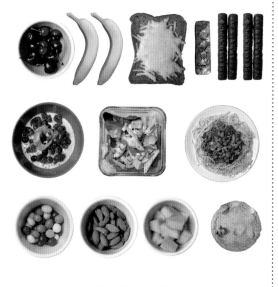

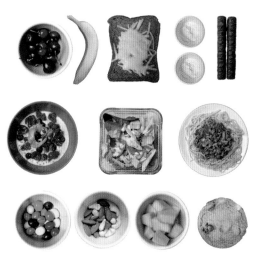

foods you enjoy

the same foods

but with fewer calories and more protein

No specific foods burn fat.

Technically, you could lose weight if you only ate chocolate bars, as long as you were in a state of calorie deficit. But chocolate bars don't contain a balance of macronutrients and have virtually no micronutrients, so your body function would not be great. And they don't contain much protein or fibre, so you're likely to feel hungry.

If you already consume enough nutritious food, it's simply a case of eating less of it. If you regularly overeat because you don't feel full, it helps to increase the amount of protein and fibre within your caloric needs to achieve fat loss.

THESE ARE ALL NUTRITIOUS FOODS BUT...

(PER 100G)

cucumber **16 cal**	pepper **23 cal**	spinach **29 cal**
broccoli **40 cal**	Brussels sprouts **42 cal**	carrots **42 cal**

semi-skimmed milk **49 cal**	0% fat Greek yogurt **54 cal**	chicken breast **105 cal**
black beans **110 cal**	turkey breast mince **112 cal**	tuna **124 cal**

quinoa **141 cal**	smoked salmon **208 cal**	honey **230 cal**
raisins **293 cal**	humous **306 cal**	dried goji berries **310 cal**

dried mango **328 cal**	1 medium avocado **350 cal**	dark chocolate **580 cal**
pistachios **585 cal**	cashews **585 cal**	peanut butter **595 cal**

You might eat a lot of natural wholefoods and wonder why you are not losing weight. Micronutrient-rich foods tend to be lower in calories than processed foods and they are rich in protein and/or fibre. But this can only be confirmed by checking the nutritional information of any given food. And, as you can see above, nutrient-dense foods can also be calorie dense because they contain fats and a lot of sugar. So you need to be mindful about the quantities you consume and ensure they are within your calorie targets for fat loss.

RIGID VS FLEXIBLE DIETS

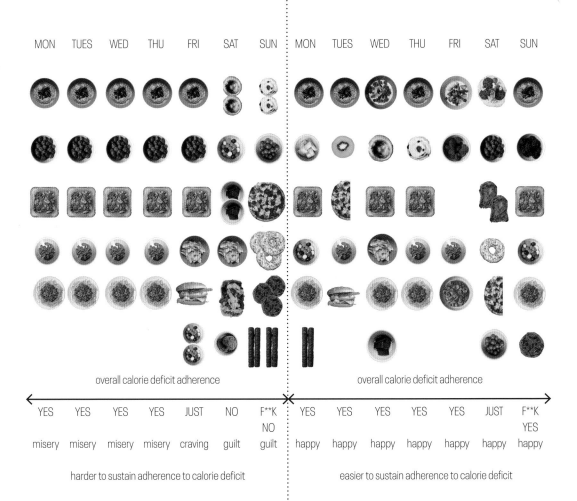

	MON	TUES	WED	THU	FRI	SAT	SUN	MON	TUES	WED	THU	FRI	SAT	SUN

overall calorie deficit adherence   overall calorie deficit adherence

YES	YES	YES	YES	JUST	NO	F**K NO	YES	YES	YES	YES	YES	JUST	F**K YES
misery	misery	misery	misery	craving	guilt	guilt	happy	happy	happy	happy	happy	happy	happy

harder to sustain adherence to calorie deficit   easier to sustain adherence to calorie deficit

If you find yourself bingeing on foods you love, it is probably because you've deprived yourself of them by following rigid dietary protocols – as the old proverb asserts, 'Absence makes the heart grow fonder'. But if these foods are regularly included in small portions, you can transform an eating schedule from uninspiring and boring into fun, enjoyable and realistic, which will increase the likelihood of calorie-deficit adherence for long periods of time.

THE FAT-LOSS TIMELINE

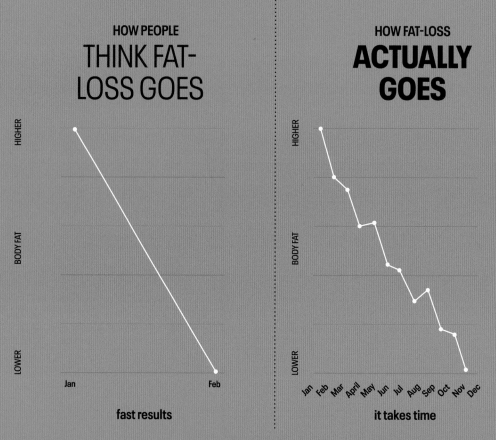

HOW PEOPLE
THINK FAT-LOSS GOES

HIGHER

BODY FAT

LOWER

Jan   Feb

fast results

HOW FAT-LOSS
ACTUALLY GOES

HIGHER

BODY FAT

LOWER

Jan Feb Mar April May Jun Jul Aug Sep Oct Nov Dec

it takes time

Just like most things in life, losing weight takes time. The weight that you want to get rid of didn't appear overnight and you need to be willing to be patient to lose it. We often set ourselves unrealistic timeframes in which to lose weight; a reflection of our incessant need for speed in all areas of modern life. Unfortunately, our physiology adapts at its own pace.

Sometimes you will stray from the calorie deficit required for fat loss, but that doesn't matter. It's what you do next that counts. Failure is never fatal because there is always a chance to continue and make progress if you really want to.

WHY CALORIE COUNTING IS NOT FOREVER

Given that calorie balance determines body composition (and you want to change body composition)

It's a good idea to appreciate calories consumed.

So that you can learn about portion size and satiety per calorie you consume.

This education will allow you to understand calories and what to eat forever after.

The idea behind counting calories is not to obsess over what you eat, but to understand the principle that will help you lose fat. Tracking calories is a temporary discipline, not a life setence. Over time, as you become more experienced, you will be able to assess portion sizes without the need to track calories.

Learning the calorie values of the food you consume could be the catalyst to finally abolishing the psychological torment you experience when you believe you are doing everything right and and yet you cannot lose weight.

Once you reach a weight you feel comfortable with, it is still important to be aware of the caloric volume you consume, but you no longer need to be in a state of caloric deficit.

THE FAT-LOSS HIERARCHY OF IMPORTANCE

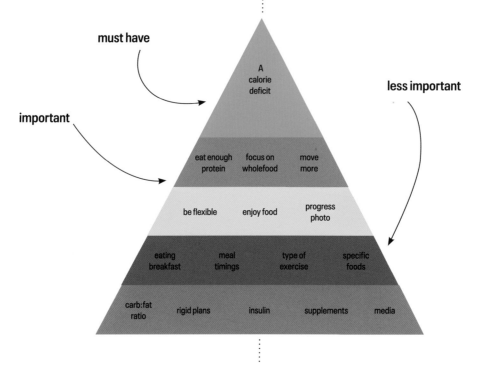

must have

important

less important

A calorie deficit

eat enough protein — focus on wholefood — move more

be flexible — enjoy food — progress photo

eating breakfast — meal timings — type of exercise — specific foods

carb:fat ratio — rigid plans — insulin — supplements — media

What we've learned so far:

A calorie deficit MUST be in place to lose weight, but it is also a good idea to focus on consuming enough protein due to its higher thermic effect/helping you feel full. And consuming enough fibre to help you feel full whilst moving more.

You don't need to waste time considering how much fat/carbs you eat, as long as they make up your overall calorie target, together with protein.

Other things that can increase your adherence to a calorie deficit are: flexibility, enjoying the food you eat, understanding portion sizes and taking progress photos instead of using scales.

Leave the bottom row for the charlatans, pseudoscientists and sensationalists to have a party with. But be sure not to turn up...

INTUITIVE EATING

LOGICAL EATING

10.30am snack:
'I fancy all of these'

680 cal

3pm snack:
'My intuition says
I require 4 of these'

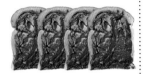

812 cal

10:30am snack:
'I like chocolate – this fits
my plan'

245 cal

3pm snack:
'I like these – and they fit
my plan'

406 cal

7pm after dinner:
'My body says these are
essential'

332 cal

7.15pm after crisps:
'If it works for Instagram
bloggers, it'll work for me'

523 cal

7pm after dinner:
'I need more nutrients and
these fit my plan'

30 cal

7.15pm after crisps:
'I like ice cream – this fits
my plan'

262 cal

2,350 cal

943 cal

Eating intuitively is entirely natural – but if
a change in body composition is the goal,
it's probably better to be aware of what
defines that change. In this case, it is
calories consumed.

The premise of intuitive eating is that it is helpful to wait for your
hunger and satiety cues before and during eating respectively. But
the potential problem with this is that while hunger is being 'dealt
with', the extent of energy you are consuming is largely unknown.
If weight loss is the aim, then this method is not usually effective.
Appreciating the number of calories you consume allows you to
calculate whether or not you're in a calorie deficit. Furthermore, this
simple, relevant knowledge stays with you for life.

FAT-LOSS FADS
TO AVOID

12 TERMS THAT MEAN NOTHING

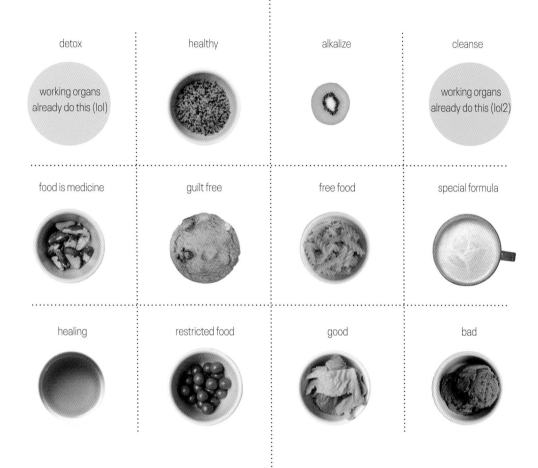

detox

working organs already do this (lol)

healthy

alkalize

cleanse

working organs already do this (lol2)

food is medicine

guilt free

free food

special formula

healing

restricted food

good

bad

We know you MUST have a calorie deficit to lose weight. But many diets, dieting strategies and slimming clubs withhold this crucial piece of information so that the consumer becomes reliant on their particular method. They also require you to make drastic changes overnight. All of the terms above are used as an alluring draw to get you to spend your hard-earned money on promises. Not one of these terms means anything scientific – therefore, when it comes to nutrition, they are extremely ambiguous. Yet they are rife in our dieting culture. You deserve better.

MEAL REPLACEMENTS

REPLACEMENT

HAPPINESS

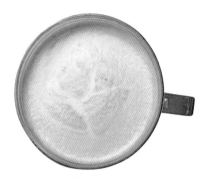

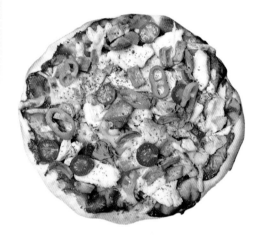

meal replacement shake sold
by a generic distributor

the f*ck meal replacements
chicken & bacon pizza

MISERY

Consume bullsh*t
Fail to understand the actual cause of your problem
Waste your money over and over again

Consume real food
Understand energy balance and nutrient consumption
Never look back

The concept of a meal replacement has no validity. You need to consume calories to remain alive, so why not do this with food? A meal replacement still contains calories, yet it promotes a dangerous message that eating food makes you fat. This simply isn't the case, as long as you understand the number of calories you eat.

A JUICE DETOX

7 DAYS ON A
JUICE DIET
FOR WEIGHT LOSS

7 DAYS ON
FOOD
FOR WEIGHT LOSS

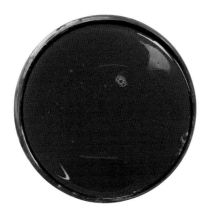

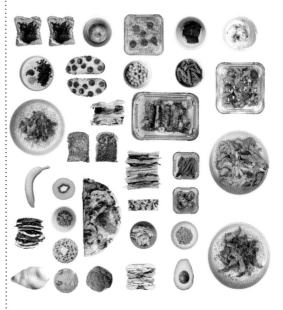

Popular – and expensive – juice diets usually last for around seven days and, unsurprisingly, deliver weight loss because of the low numbers of calories consumed.

Some argue that a juice diet will 'kick-start' weight loss. But once you have lost weight over seven days, the chance of that weight returning is highly likely, given that you haven't learned during your juice fast how to maintain this weight loss while eating food afterwards.

You will lose weight for the long term if you avoid juice diets and begin making pragmatic caloric adjustments to your existing diet.

SLIMMING CLUBS

SLIMMING CLUBS

RESTRICTED FOOD

CALORIE DEFICIT

FOOD AND DRINKS

'EAT AS MUCH AS YOU LIKE'

TRACK CALORIES

gain 1lb	lose 1lb	gain 2lbs

'I'm failing'	'I'm succeeding'	'I'm failing again'

scales don't measure fat loss

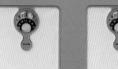

move more	track calories	take photos
	EAT FEWER CALORIES THAN YOU EXPEND	
enjoyment	informed	see progress

Complicated
an unnecessary way to think about food and fat loss

Educated
a rational and objective way to approach food and fat loss

Despite their supporters, there are many reasons why the approach taken by slimming clubs may not support your fat-loss goal:

1. The win or lose arena
Success/failure is determined each week by a weigh-in. In view of daily weight fluctuations, this is an inaccurate method to measure weekly fat-loss progress.

2. Good and bad foods
Food type does not directly determine fat loss, but quantity does. Yet slimming clubs label foods as good or bad based on point systems and complicated methodology. These terms can conjure feelings of shame that wreaks havoc on your relationship with food.

3. Free foods
Unlimited consumption of a selection of foods (some of which are calorie dense) very easily creates a caloric surplus even while following strict 'free food' protocols.

4. Failure to address energy balance (caloric deficit)
The withholding of the most critical piece of fat-loss information is strategically designed to create the notion that only the slimming club's formula can help you.

For some, slimming clubs do work. But, if addressed scientifically, this is down to the physiological principles of negative energy balance over time, not by adhering to free foods, smart points or speed foods.

Once you realize that fat loss needs you to address your energy balance, then you forego any sense of guilt, shame and confusion, and replace it with an informed, lifelong education.

DIET PILLS
& DIET TEAS

SPENDING
YOUR MONEY
ON STARVING YOURSELF

SPENDING
YOUR MONEY
ON EATING FOOD YOU LIKE

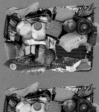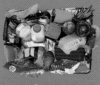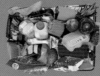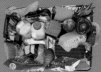

28 DAYS' WORTH OF
APPETITE SUPPRESSANTS
AS ENDORSED BY
SOCIAL MEDIA
CELEBRITIES

28 DAYS' WORTH OF FOOD

£119.99
money spent on unproven promises

£119.99
money spent on food, to be eaten as part of
an informed and sustainable lifestyle.

Diet pills, teas and other products directly contribute to disordered
eating and unnecessary fear of food. Many people believe the
unsubstantiated claims of their favourite social-media influencer and
spend hard-earned money on these products. Please spend your
money on actual food and enjoy eating it within your calorie targets.

THE INTERNET VS THE REAL WORLD

THE INTERNET

THE REALITY

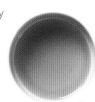

'Green tea boosts metabolism.'

'Green tea eliminates cellulite.'

No more than any other drink.

No it doesn't. And what's wrong with cellulite?

'Green tea burns body fat.'

'Green tea detoxifies your body.'

A calorie deficit reduces fat.

No it doesn't, you have organs that do that.

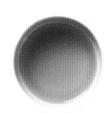

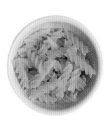

'Refined carbs make you fat.'

'Carbs spike insulin, which is bad.'

A calorie surplus makes you fat.

So does protein. And it aids fat loss.

'Refined carbs are high GI, which is bad.'

'Carbs make you diabetic.'

The glycaemic index (GI) is an anecdote.

Billions disprove this.

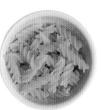

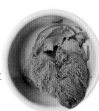

'You should never eat saturated fat.'

'Sugar is poison.'

It has low GI – by this logic we should eat lots of it.

Then all fruit is poison – yet it is not.

'Stop promoting junk food and misleading people.'

'You should feel guilty eating ice cream.'

People are intelligent enough to interpret the facts.

No food should make you feel guilty, ever.

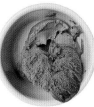

Despite the well-documented, heavily endorsed and believable viability of some nutritional claims, no elixirs exist that can transform your health singlehandedly. And, despite the paid ads that appear at the top of the internet's search results, there is no miracle.

We need to be aware and vigilant to identify unsubstantiated, biased, misleading information, and to dismiss it as insignificant.

THE PROBLEM WITH THE DIETING INDUSTRY

When you get a flat tyre, you ask a reputable garage for a new one in exchange for money. But if you imagine obesity as a flat tyre, most diet companies take your money but knowingly give you another flat tyre in return. Like any business, companies in the dieting industry exist to make money.

Such companies promote the false perception (and hope) that rapid weight loss and supplements are necessary. They do not encourage practicality or a sustainable, gradual, measured approach.

A quick internet search brings up a plethora of well-marketed, rapid weight-loss solutions, supplements and diet plans. In hope and expectation, these are the solutions people choose. Yet the connection between net spend on such products and the global obesity rate clearly shows that instead of solving the problem, they perpetuate it.

This said, fad diets are not to blame for increasing global obesity rates. The bottom line is that we consume too many calories and do not move enough.

We make our own choices, and if we want to succeed we should consult evidence-based information. Change requires knowledge, education and, above all, consistency. You do not need a new diet. You just need to understand (and then adjust) the one you already have. This will cost you £0 and change your life forever.

WHAT IS MARKETED

GET
SLIM
COFFEE

coffee that makes
you sh*t yourself

CLEANSING
TEA DETOX

tea that makes you
sh*t yourself

CURB YOUR
CRAVINGS
LOL

appetite-reducing
shots made of ?

STOP EATING
REAL FOOD
& DRINK ME

meal
replacements full
of calories anyway

BCAAs

BCAAs, as used
by a model
or influencer

FAT
METABOLIZER

pills that defy 7
billion years of
human evolution

I'M RIPPING
YOU OFF

a juice detox
because your
working organs
are on holiday

FAT
BURNER
PILLS

magical fat
burners that are
merely caffeine

DON'T EAT!
'AVE A LOLLIPOP
INSTEAD

appetite-
suppressant
lollipop that
contains the
same calories as a
regular lollipop

£1,008.95

items that make no meaningful
changes to your health

WHAT IS IGNORED

real food

education

empathy

energy balance

evidence

moderation

enjoyment

nutrients

nutrients

honesty

£27.55

real food with energy and nutrients to remain alive

FAT-LOSS MYTHS
TO FORGET

NUTRITION MYTHS
OF THE PAST 30 YEARS

'Carbs make you fat'

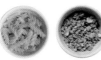

evidence: ?

'Low carb is best for fat loss'

evidence: ?

'Sugar makes you fat'

evidence: ?

'Keto is the best way to lose fat'

evidence: ?

'Intermittent fasting is best for fat loss'

evidence: ?

'Starvation mode exists and makes you fat'

evidence: ?

'Eating clean will help you lose weight'

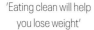

evidence: ?

'Eating any fast food makes you fat and unhealthy'

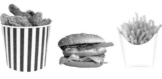

evidence: ?

'Fat makes you fat'

evidence: ?

These claims still exist because we want to believe them. Our challenge is to forego the impulse to believe these extravagant claims and put our trust in the actual evidence.

Today, a presentation on nutrition advice for optimal health would require 842 Powerpoint slides and a martian to present it. Everything we see or hear is a contradiction and the result is a toxic dieting culture full of ridicule, self-righteousness and confusion.

- Millions of people outlaw food groups that they have been told can individually cause fat gain. Yet there is no reference to actual science.

- Documentaries share wild accusations about foods and biased opinion rather than sharing facts.

- People we consider trusted experts claim sugar is the sole cause of obesity, labelling it as poison, which is unsubstantiated opinion.

- Studies on rats are put forward as evidence of impact on human bodies, yet we are not rats.

- There is no context anymore – not for individuals who seek rational guidance on a very simple nutritional goal. Instead, they face exhaustion from irrelevant fear-mongering and a bottomless pit of disappointing chaos, resulting in the curtailment of their goals.

YOU have the power to educate yourself and question motives and contexts.

You can choose to accept information or throw it into the multi-billion pound landfill where the majority of the dieting industry should reside.

MYTH 1:
CARBS MAKE YOU FAT

Because fruit and vegetables
are mostly carbs...

Because these sources of 'carbs' contain other
macronutrients, such as fat...

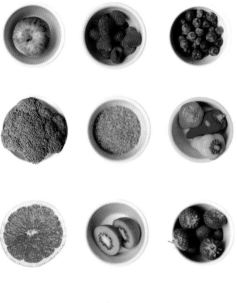

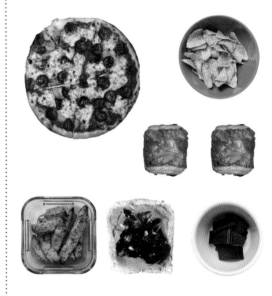

... they are
low in calories

... they are
high in calories

It's a good idea to correctly differentiate the food before trying to demonize it. Overall calorie balance will define fat loss, not carbs. Over the past 30 years or so the consumption of carbs has been villified by those who believe that carbs impact on body fat more than any other macronutrient. The examples displayed on the right of this graphic represent foods that contain calories from carbs, protein and, more pertinently, fat. And fruit and vegetables are mostly made up of carbohydrates. 'Does broccoli make you fat?'

MYTH 2:
LOW CARB IS BEST FOR FAT LOSS

low carb   low fat

The rate of fat loss is the same in both. Total calories in vs calories out is what matters for fat loss/maintenance/gain – not carbs or fat.

One meta-analysis* undertaken in 2018 by Hall & Guo found that the rates of fat loss on low-carb or low-fat diets were virtually the same when calories and protein were equated. In fact, low-fat diets showed a slightly greater amount of fat loss, but the difference was too negligible to be significant.

*Meta-analysis and systematic reviews are reliable, unbiased ways to determine conclusions because they review all relevant scientific research, whereas a single study may have biased conditions or tell only half the story.

MYTH 3:
SUGAR MAKES YOU FAT

100g sugar

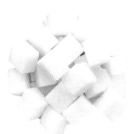

100g sugar within food

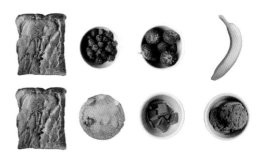

400 cal

1,308 cal

Despite what you've heard, sugar is not bad. We just like to blame an easy target for our problems.

Sugar is a simple carbohydrate found in many natural foods, such as fruit, and in processed foods, such as cake. Eaten on its own, it is digested quickly compared to a complex carbohydrate, such as grains. This is because complex carbs contain fibre and pure sugar contains no fibre. As we know, fibre also fills you up for longer and is good for body function.

100g of refined pure sugar amounts to 400 calories. The sweet foods on the right also contain 100g of sugar, but their total calories equal 1,308 calories. That is because 908 non-sugar related calories exist within these foods. This is more relevant to body composition.

Eating high volumes of sugar-rich foods lacking in protein and fibre may contribute to becoming overweight, but only because you are likely to eat more of them as your body will digest them faster and burn fewer calories while doing so (remember protein burns more calories during digestion).

'I CUT OUT REFINED SUGAR
AND LOST WEIGHT'

60g iced doughnut	500ml tub of peanut butter cup ice cream	40g chocolate chip cookie
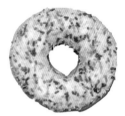	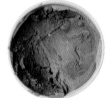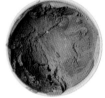	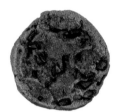
248 cal	**1,400 cal**	**188 cal**

calories from sugar	calories from other carbs, protein & fat	calories from sugar	calories from other carbs, protein & fat	calories from sugar	calories from other carbs, protein & fat
32 cal	**216 cal**	420 cal	**980 cal**	64 cal	**124 cal**
13% of total calories	**87% of total calories**	30% of total calories	**70% of total calories**	34% of total calories	**66% of total calories**

There is a misconception that the rise in type II diabetes has correlated with a rise in sugar consumption over the last 30 years. But while we are eating more sugar, sugar is not the main cause of type II diabetes – being overweight, having significant abdominal fat and genetics are.

Visceral fat around organs may begin to affect the ability of the pancreas to secrete insulin into the bloodstream and regulate blood sugar after consuming calories. (Insulin is a hormone that regulates movement of sugar into cells and lowers sugar in the bloodstream.) Eventually, the pancreas reaches a point where it can no longer function properly or produce enough insulin to regulate blood sugar properly and type II diabetes is diagnosed. Thereafter, consumption of sugar-dense foods and drinks and large meals can become problematic as blood sugar cannot be regulated as well.

But it is possible to reverse type II diabetes, mainly by simply losing weight via a calorie deficit.

MYTH 4:
KETO IS BEST FOR FAT LOSS

KETO	CARBS
friendly foods for fat loss	not allowed on the keto diet

bulletproof coffee	7 rashers of streaky bacon	75g almonds	hot chocolate	90g bagel	100g blueberries
480 cal	270 cal	455 cal	188 cal	232 cal	68 cal

50g grass-fed butter	keto carbonara	1 large avocado	150g cooked rice	pasta carbonara	150g banana
375 cal	816 cal	350 cal	239 cal	611 cal	135 cal

2,746 cal   **1,473 cal**

Keto claims to burn more fat than other dieting methods – but that is simply because more fat is consumed.

For fat loss, it is total calories that count. If you enjoy carbs, you can absolutely include them in any dieting goal.

The ketogenic diet was invented as a clinical intervention to stop seizures in epileptic children. It works by inducing ketosis, a metabolic state in which the body converts fat into compounds called ketones and uses them for energy. Over the years it seems to have morphed into a weight-loss concept, whereby you eat more fat and fewer carbs. The irony is that the foods keto zealots claim are vital for fat loss can actually be much higher in calories than those they forbid because they are too high in carbs.

The claim is that eliminating carbs and eating large amounts of dietary fat instead results in more total fat burned. But you simply burn the dietary fat consumed, not more total body fat.

Many keto lovers believe that secretion of insulin defines body fat, but while it is involved in the role of converting energy into body fat, it does not define it. Total body fat will always be governed by total calories in vs calories out inclusive of any ratio of consumed macronutrients.

MYTH 5:
INTERMITTENT FASTING
IS BEST FOR FAT LOSS

intermittent fasting
for fat loss

8-hour feeding window

usually between 10am & 6pm

2,000 calories
consumed over 8 hours

eating when you want
for fat loss

eat in the morning...

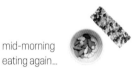

mid-morning eating again...

hungry at lunch so eating...

post-workout eating...

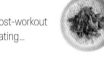
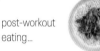

dinner and socializing...

feeling hungry eating a snack at night...

2,000 calories
consumed in the course of a whole day

Intermittent fasting is a popular fat-loss strategy. In this '16:8' example, an individual fasts for 16 hours (sleeping during this time), leaving an 8-hour window to eat a day's worth of food. Research suggests that intermittent fasting can result in fat loss, but this is because the fasters simply reduced their calorie intake. Intermittent fasting helps some people eat within their calorie deficit, while others find it too difficult. Do what works for you.

MYTH 6:
STARVATION MODE EXISTS?

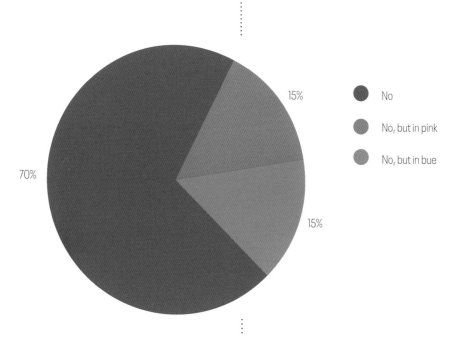

70%

15%

15%

- ⬤ No
- ⬤ No, but in pink
- ⬤ No, but in bue

Despite claims, your body does not go into 'starvation mode' and prevent you from burning fat. If you have gained fat or your fat-loss progress has stalled, it's because you are no longer in a calorie deficit as a result of one or more of the following:

1. You are underestimating how many calories you're actually eating (for example, you think it's 1,200 but it's actually 1,700).
2. The amount you move or exercise has been reduced because you have less energy, meaning that you burn fewer calories.
3. Metabolic adaptation – after a period of aggressive caloric deficit, metabolism adapts so that resting energy expenditure is less than before, meaning you aren't burning the number of calories expected at rest.
4. As your weight reduces on a calorie deficit, you did not continue to reduce calories or increase energy expenditure to stay in a calorie deficit.

MYTH 7:
EATING CLEAN WILL HELP
YOU LOSE WEIGHT

STEP 1:
select and unwrap your 'dirty' food

STEP 2:
wash food thouroughly until 'clean'

STEP 3:
dry off cleansed food and consume

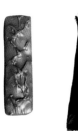

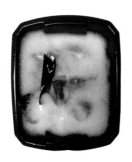

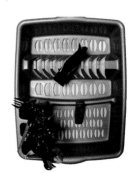

Oh, you meant these? Well, these are not 'clean' foods. Scientifically, they are just foods with more micronutrients than others.

The term 'clean eating' has no scientific meaning when it comes to fat loss; it tells us nothing useful or measurable. But the problem with this term is that if there is a 'clean', there must be a 'dirty', which also means nothing useful or measurable about the food, apart from the fact that it has been demonized.

All food still contains calories. By idolizing some foods (including raw and alkaline foods) and demonizing others, the clean-eating brigade are confusing the functional benefits of consuming nutrients with energy balance, which is what determines fat loss.

'SUPERFOOD'

JUST FOOD

50g dried goji berries

100g strawberries

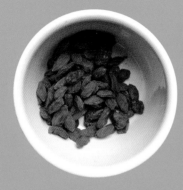

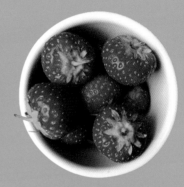

155 cal
25g sugar
not so super...

30 cal
6g sugar

There is no such thing as a superfood; it is simply a food dense in nutrients. The 'superfood' label may lead you to think you can consume copious amounts, but, as you can see here, some so-called superfoods are calorie dense in comparison with foods not so lucky as to have been chosen by the superfood selection panel, but still nutrient dense and relatively low in calories.

MYTH 8: EATING FAST FOOD MAKES YOU FAT

'MAKES YOU THIN'

100g fruit & nut mix

500ml
super smoothie

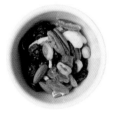

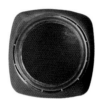

503 cal
10g protein

302 cal
50g sugar
0g fibre

805 cal

'MAKES YOU FAT'

9 fast food
chicken nuggets

500ml coke

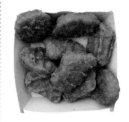

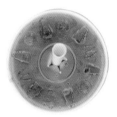

388 cal
24g protein

210 cal
53g sugar
0g fibre

598 cal

This is not a competition so much as a factual illustration. A large handful of fruit-and-nut mix with a health-branded smoothie serve as a nutritious snack, which many think will benefit their weight. Yet, a portion of chicken nuggets and a large coke is viewed as a terrible choice that will make you fat, but this 'fast food' option has significantly fewer calories and more protein. You can eat 'fast food' and lose weight as long as you consume it within your daily targets and understand that you should still focus on wholefoods most of the time.

FOOD:
PERCEPTION VS REALITY

MYTH 9:
FAT MAKES YOU FAT

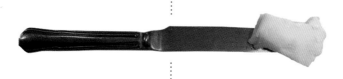

In the '90s, fat was heavily demonized and labelled as the culprit that made us overweight. This isn't surprising given that its calorie volume per gram is more than double that of protein and carbs (see page 24). But like protein and carbs, there is no evidence anywhere to suggest that any one macronutrient stores fat more than another.

Consuming large quantities of fat may contribute to being overweight given the caloric volume included in relatively small amounts of fat-rich foods, but be sure to know that fat as a macronutrient is not the direct cause.

A lot of the calorie-saving alternatives you see reduce the amount of fat in their product because fat is calorie dense, not because fat is bad.

It is a good idea to look further than the 'reduced fat' or 'low fat' labels on food packaging to see calorie and macronutrient amounts, free from marketing agendas. 'Low calorie' is a more useful label.

Some fats benefit our health, such as mono/polyunsaturated fats found in fish, nuts, avocado and seeds. Others, such as saturated fat found in butter, coconut oil, dairy products and animal fat don't provide any specific benefit to functional health, but offer other nutritional benefits, taste good, and should be eaten in moderation.

The only cause of weight gain is simply consuming more total calories than you expend consistently over time, not eating fat.

1,000 CALORIES

1,000 CALORIES

25 strawberries, 143 blueberries, 100g chicken breast,
110g tuna steak, 3 apricots, 100g kidney beans, 100g cantaloupe
melon, 3 mini peppers, 100g cherries, 100g brocclli,
½ cucumber, 20g mixed seeds

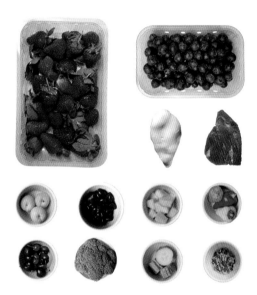

20g mixed seeds	250g fillet steak	17 Brazil nuts (or 75g)

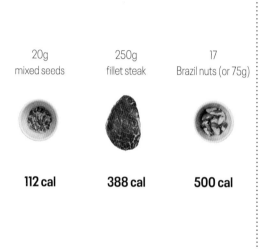

112 cal	**388 cal**	**500 cal**

1,000 calories can look very different. Just because the volume of
food is small, it doesn't mean that you aren't consuming a relatively
large number of calories. Use a calorie calculator to check calories
per weight of foods. You'd be amazed how much of certain foods
you can eat and how many calories are in some of your favourite
'health' foods because they are nutrient- and calorie-dense.

I'M LOSING WEIGHT BUT EATING MORE THAN EVER

20ml olive oil, 20ml coconut oil,
30g peanut butter & 3 chocolates

600g of strawberries

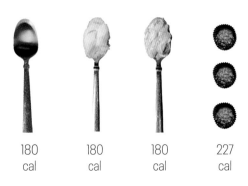

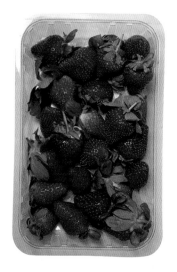

| 180 cal | 180 cal | 180 cal | 227 cal |

767 cal

low volume | high calories

180 cal

high volume | low calories

By consuming a greater volume of low-calorie foods, but fewer
calories than before, you will be able to lose weight but eat more.

You can easily reduce the calories you eat while increasing the
volume of food you eat and lose weight. But remember that this
isn't because you're 'stoking your metabolic furnace', it's just
because the foods you've selected are lower in calories. If you were
used to eating large amounts of food before, it makes sense to
continue to consume relatively large amounts of low-calorie food
so that you feel full and still meet your calorie deficit needs. Fruits
and vegetables exist to champion this target.

'HEALTHY COOKING'

ALSO COOKING

15ml olive/coconut oil for 365 meals per year

A non-stick pan for 365 meals per year

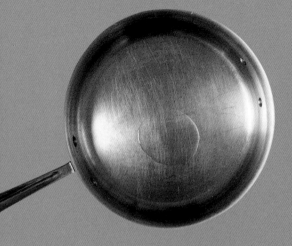

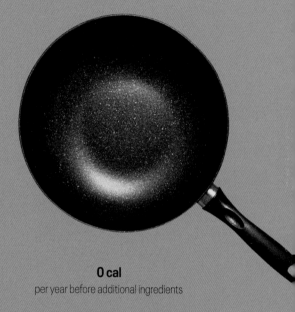

49,275 cal

0 cal

per year before additional ingredients

per year before additional ingredients

49,275 calories equates to approximately 6.3kg (1st or 14lb) of body fat.
Over time, consistent small changes can have a big overall impact.

Using 15ml of olive oil per day for cooking purposes will result in the consumption of beneficial monounsaturated fats, but also 135 calories. Over a calendar year, that equates to 49,275 calories before any additional ingredients – and approximately 6.3kg/1 stone in body weight.

If lubrication is the sole reason for using oils to cook with, a non-stick pan offers an opportunity to reduce body weight by 6.3kg/1 stone in a calendar year, or free up calories to be consumed elsewhere. This saving of 135 calories each day offers a significant chance, over time, to reduce overall calorie intake with minimal sacrifice. Small changes can reap big rewards.

'HEALTHY'

kiwi & strawberry flavoured water

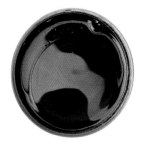

120 cal

32g sugar | 0g fibre

contains vitamins

FORGOTTEN

Any amount of water, a fresh kiwi
and 100g of real strawberries

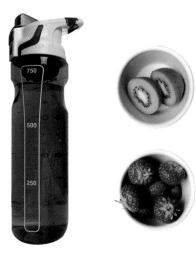

69 cal

13g sugar | 3g fibre
(and you get to eat)

also contains vitamins

The attraction to vitamin-enriched 'healthy' water may be that it offers you micronutrients and hydration at the same time. But they also offer you added calories. If a vitamin-enriched water, for example, contains 120 calories, those calories are mainly derived from sugar.

By comparison, you could achieve the same hydration by drinking water, and you could eat 100g of strawberries and a kiwi fruit for approximately half the calories of the 'healthy' water. You would also consume more fibre.

THE PROTEIN PROBLEM

WITH MARKETING   **WITHOUT** MARKETING

1 x protein cereal bar	28g veggie protein nut mix	360ml berry 'protein' smoothie	50g slice of generic bread	28g salted peanuts	360ml semi-skimmed milk

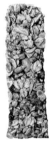   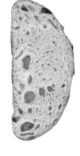 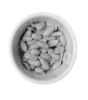

4g protein	**7g protein**	**8g protein**	**5g protein**	**8g protein**	**13g protein**
123 cal	130 cal	212 cal	95 cal	171 cal	180 cal
6g sugar	1g sugar	33g sugar	2g sugar	1g sugar	17g sugar

You may want to compare protein quantities with other relevant nutritional variables and the price before choosing...

Protein is beneficial to most dieting goals, not least weight loss and brands have created 'protein' versions of new or existing products to appeal to those who choose a high-protein diet. But the word 'protein' on the packaging doesn't mean it's the right choice for you. For example, for a typical 30g serving of protein from the smoothie protein drink, you'd have to consume four of them – more than 800 calories. If you opt for the 'healthy' protein bar, you would consume less protein and more calories than a slice of bread contains. Protein is essential, but there's no need to source it from portions promoted by brands to cash in on a beneficial macronutrient. Instead, consider cheaper sources without exaggerated headlines.

WHICH PROTEIN POWDER IS BEST?

TUBES OF TOOTHPASTE

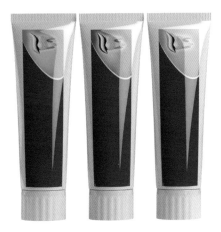

PROTEIN POWDER

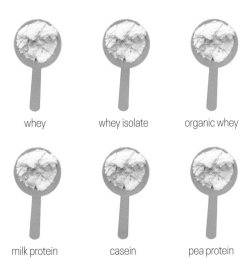

whey   whey isolate   organic whey

milk protein   casein   pea protein

despite the range of products
ALL CLEAN YOUR TEETH
It doesn't matter what you choose

despite the range of products
ALL ARE A SCOOP OF PROTEIN
It also doesn't matter what you choose

Whey protein is simply a waste product of milk often used in shakes, but there are also several other versions of protein powder available that do exactly the same job as whey. Supplement companies encourage you to buy different types of whey protein, claiming each contain standalone benefits, but as all toothpastes clean your teeth, most protein powders have an identical effect. In the same way that all toothpastes clean your teeth, in most instances casein protein will have the same effect as whey or whey isolate. If you want to conveniently add protein powder to your shakes, yogurt or porridge, just choose the cheapest version.

HOW TO IMPROVE YOUR RELATIONSHIP WITH FOOD

EMOTION	SCIENCE

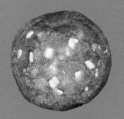 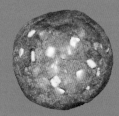

| 'This cookie is junk food and eating it will make me fat.' | **240 calories.** Minimal micronutrients, but tasty as a treat. |

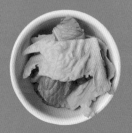 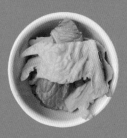

| 'Eating this lettuce is good and will make me thin.' | No. An overall calorie deficit will result in fat loss. |

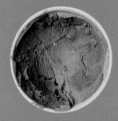 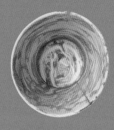

| 'I've been bad and have ruined all my progress. I may as well eat this whole tub of ice cream.' | No. You consumed 150 enjoyable calories. Then you consumed another 1,000 calories through guilt. Eating the whole tub is the part that ruined your calorie deficit. |

Emotion does not control your nutritional wellbeing – science does.

Science is objective; emotion is subjective. Science helps you learn about the relevance of nutrition; emotion is useless in this respect.

Next time you are about to lambast yourself for eating a cookie or some ice cream, remind yourself that understanding the nutritional facts will be more useful than beating yourself up. That way, you'll appreciate that any food can be eaten.

HOW TO IMPROVE YOUR RELATIONSHIP WITH FOOD

EMOTIONAL
OVER-EATING

A PROBLEM OCCURS:
Four cinnamon swirls:
'I need these.'

A PROBLEM OCCURS:
Confront problem:
'Four cinnamon swirls do not solve my problem.'

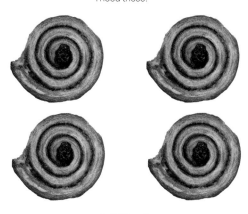

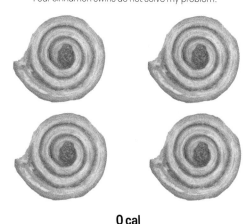

1,460 cal
(and still have an unsolved problem)

0 cal
(and have a solved problem)

You will always have the power of conscious thought to decide
what, where and why you consume food. Food will never control
you. You will always control it – remember that.

Whatever therapy or treatment you embark on to combat
emotional/binge eating, if it is successful, it will result in you
explicitly deciding NOT to emotionally overeat. But, here's the thing
– you already have the power to do that now. We have normalized
the idea the food can control us. All this does is give a subconscious
excuse for its perpetual hold over you.

Events in your life can cause pain and suffering, but your intelligence
will always tell you that food has no bearing on healing or solving
these problems. You have 100 per cent control over your nutritional
decisions in times of stress. The simplicity of yes or no is there if you
allow it to be.

HOW TO IMPROVE YOUR RELATIONSHIP WITH FOOD

WHAT HAPPENS WHEN YOU EAT A PIZZA

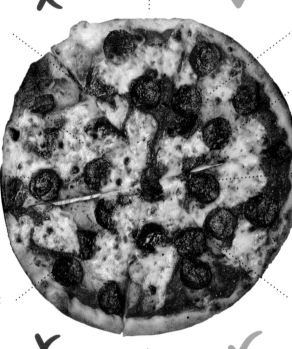

✗   ✓

'I just gained a stone.'

You didn't gain a stone.

'I ruined ALL of my progress.'

You didn't ruin ANY of your progress.

'I love pizza but I hereby BAN it forever!'

You CAN fit pizza into your calorie intake. Simply adjust the rest of your day/week.

You were going to eat a meal anyway, this one had a few extra calories. That is it.

'I may as well give up and eat the contents of my fridge.'

✗   ✓

The same applies for any calorie-dense food.

When you eat pizza, you experience the same metabolic process as you would if you ate any food. It enters first the stomach, then the gastrointestinal tract where nutrients are absorbed and passed into the bloodstream. Pizza (or any calorie-dense food) simply has a greater caloric density when this digestion takes place – but the process is the same.

The potential for damage that one pizza has on your health is entirely dependent on your psychological state when or after consuming it, not its ingredients.

FEAR

POWER

THE FEAR THEY SPREAD:

HOW YOU ANSWER THEM:

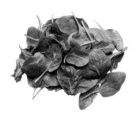 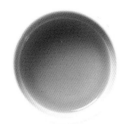 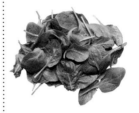 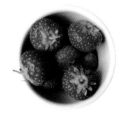

'You MUST eat nutrient-dense wholefoods ALL the time or you'll DIE.'

'You MUST drink this cleansing tea because you'll lose weight and rid yourself of toxins that will KILL you.'

Stop being a berk. I eat them because they optimize my functional health.

Thanks, but I have a working liver and I'd prefer to consume food.

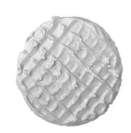 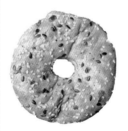 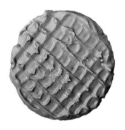

'You CAN'T eat this bagel because your body doesn't know how to PROCESS it.'

'You CANNOT eat biscuits because they cause inflammation and DISEASE.'

Be quiet. Of course my body knows how to process macronutrients.

Overall lifestyle and genetics influence those things. Not one biscuit.

Succumbing to those who create fear via pseudoscience in order to sell you something.

Being armed with the power to ignore nutritional propaganda designed to take your food freedom away.

No individual food can have an extreme outcome on your weight. Therefore, you don't need to be protected from it. Instead, you need to be informed. The critical element important to your overall health regarding food is the regularity and quantities in which you consume food. If any of us drank too much water, we would die.

But if we drink an adequate amount to stay hydrated, we will not. If an individual eats too many biscuits, it could be problematic. But eating a number of biscuits or any enjoyed food as part of a varied, calorie-controlled diet, balanced in all macronutrients means that eating those foods is not problematic.

It is only when you remove the fear you have absorbed from scare-mongering rhetoric that you have the power to make your own informed decisions and understand more about the food you eat and its true effect on your body.

'EATING HEALTHILY'

BEING INFORMED

'These almonds are a better snack than chocolate and will help you lose weight because chocolate is bad.'

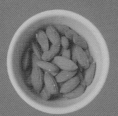

'This is 75g of almonds. Almonds contain micronutrients and antioxidants. But this amount is still 460 calories – double the average chocolate bar.'

'These blackberries are a must-have inclusion in your diet because they're super healthy.'

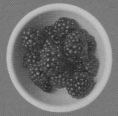

'This is 100g of blackberries. They are rich in many micronutrients and fibre. They are low in calories, but you don't have to eat them...'

'OMG you have to eat goji berries if you want to be healthy and lose weight. They are a superfood, after all.'

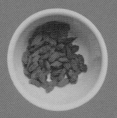

'50g of dried goji berries contains 155 calories and 25g of sugar – similar to 50g of fruit gums. I'm choosing the fruit gums this time as a moderated treat because they can be included in an overall diet that still supports my goals.'

Information sourced from a clickbait blog.

Information sourced from factual information and rational thought processes.

The word 'healthy' means absolutely nothing useful. Instead, understanding the caloric and approximate macronutrient, fibre and micronutrient values of the food you eat arms you with information that is useful. This way you are empowered to make supportive choices and still enjoy everything you eat.

WORTHLESS
TERMS

✗

'This meal is
healthy.'

'This meal is
unhealthy.'

'This meal is
good.'

'This meal is
bad.'

'This meal is
nourishing.'

'This meal is
guilt-free.'

'This meal is
a cheat.'

WORTHFUL
FACTS

✓

'This meal has many
nutrients.'

'This meal has
few nutrients.'

'This meal is
supportive.'

'This meal is
not supportive.'

'This meal is
balanced.'

'This meal is
low in calories.'

'This meal is
high in calories.'

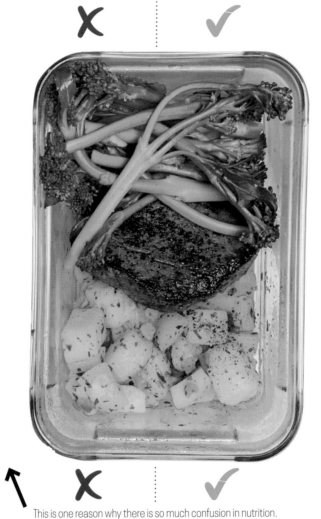

✗ ✓

This is one reason why there is so much confusion in nutrition.

The amount of worthless jargon circulating in dieting spheres is enough to completely ruin your understanding of basic nutrition. The terms on the left mean nothing useful and spoil the actual meanings on the right, which communicate directly with factors that are relevant to your goal.

TRYING

yum

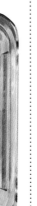

THEM:
'You're seriously going to eat that shite?'
YOU:
'Oh...'

TRYING

is this better?

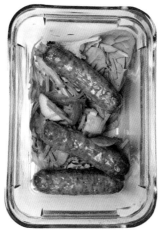

THEM:
'On a health kick are we? (smirk)'
YOU:
'Oh...'

TRYING AGAIN

surely now?

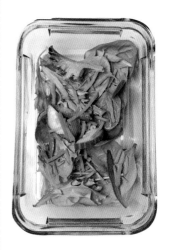

THEM:
'God, that looks plain and dry'
YOU:
'I give up.'

You just can't win these days... Don't let others ridicule your nutritional journey based on their own vindictiveness or lack of knowledge.

Choose carefully who you listen to. You can remove the vindictive noise from your life if you surround yourself with practical, evidence-based principles. Ignore those people in the office who, after watching another agenda-driven TV programme about nutrition, continue to inflict its exaggerated inaccuracies on you when you're just trying to eat your f*cking lunch. Put their keyboard in the bin.

HOW TO ENJOY
BREAKFAST

A lot has been written about breakfast over the years: breakfast 'is the most important meal of the day for fat loss', 'kick-starts your metabolism for fat loss' and, most recently, by intermittent fasters: 'skipping breakfast supports fat loss'.

Yet, if we address these claims with the latest hard evidence, we can conclude that the facts are:

- Breakfast is just one of many meals eaten throughout the day.

- Every meal is important for fat loss.

- Breakfast is not the only meal that 'kick-starts' our metabolism. Whenever we eat food, we metabolize food.

The only thing that is different about breakfast, compared with other meals in the day, is that it is usually the first meal that comes after a long break from eating and, thus, the first opportunity to acquire energy after you wake.

Skipping breakfast is not automatically going to result in more fat loss. But it may help you eat fewer calories, as long as you don't go wild with lunch, dinner and the snacks in between.

Ultimately, total calories in compared with total calories out over days, weeks and months determines fat loss, not whether or not you eat breakfast.

If you prefer eating breakfast, eat it. If you prefer skipping breakfast, skip it.

'GOOD'

2 tsp acai powder,
50g frozen blueberries,
150g greek yogurt,
2 bananas, 30g granola,
40g peanut butter,
20g dessicated coconut,
15g cacao nibs, 10g linseed,
10g flaxseeed, 5g chia seeds

1,057 cal
34g protein
contains a lot of nutrients
**and probably excessive
calories/sugar**

'BAD'

3 bacon rashers, 1 egg,
2 pork sausages, 1 tomato,
30g mushrooms, handful
spinach & 10ml olive oil

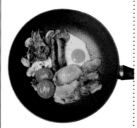

531 cal
40g protein
contains moderate calories/
sugar **and probably enough
nutrients**

'FAT-LOSS' FOOD

100g fruit
& nut granola

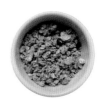

350 cal
10g protein
with nutrients and fibre

'FAT-GAIN' FOOD

100g iced
cinnamon bun

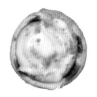

350 cal
8g protein
with fewer nutrients and fibre

'CLEAN'

75g fruit & nut granola, 150g
0% fat Greek yogurt, 20g
goji berries, 10g desiccated
coconut, 1 banana, 20g
linseed, 10g chia seeds,
250ml fruit juice

929 cal
28g protein

'DIRTY'

Bacon & egg muffin
+ hash brown

484 cal
22g protein

'GOOD'

50g red berries cereal
+ 200ml skimmed milk

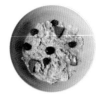

288 cal
11g protein

'BAD'

50g choco pops
+ 200ml skimmed milk

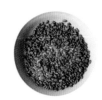

291 cal
11g protein

There is no good, bad, fat-loss, fat-gain, clean or dirty breakfast.
Smoothie or granola bowls may be a solid source of micronutrients,
but do consider their caloric density and sugar content if you are
trying to lose weight. A fry-up can be lower in calories (and, being
higher in protein, may keep you fuller for longer).

CEREAL

(per 50g with 200ml semi-skimmed milk)

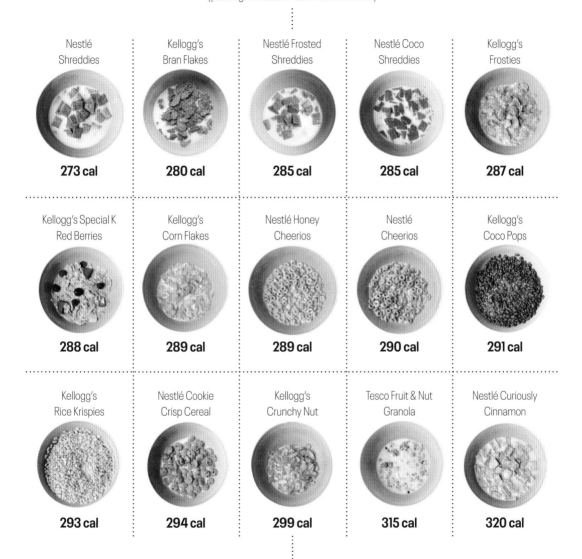

Nestlé Shreddies	Kellogg's Bran Flakes	Nestlé Frosted Shreddies	Nestlé Coco Shreddies	Kellogg's Frosties
273 cal	**280** cal	**285** cal	**285** cal	**287** cal
Kellogg's Special K Red Berries	Kellogg's Corn Flakes	Nestlé Honey Cheerios	Nestlé Cheerios	Kellogg's Coco Pops
288 cal	**289** cal	**289** cal	**290** cal	**291** cal
Kellogg's Rice Krispies	Nestlé Cookie Crisp Cereal	Kellogg's Crunchy Nut	Tesco Fruit & Nut Granola	Nestlé Curiously Cinnamon
293 cal	**294** cal	**299** cal	**315** cal	**320** cal

Cereals are often demonized by those limiting their calories but even brands without the healthy marketing enjoyed by granola or 'healthy' cereals can contain similar amounts of protein and fibre, and often less sugar and fewer calories. Be aware that 'healthy' foods might not be doing you any favours when it comes to losing weight – check their calorie content.

MILK

(per 200ml)

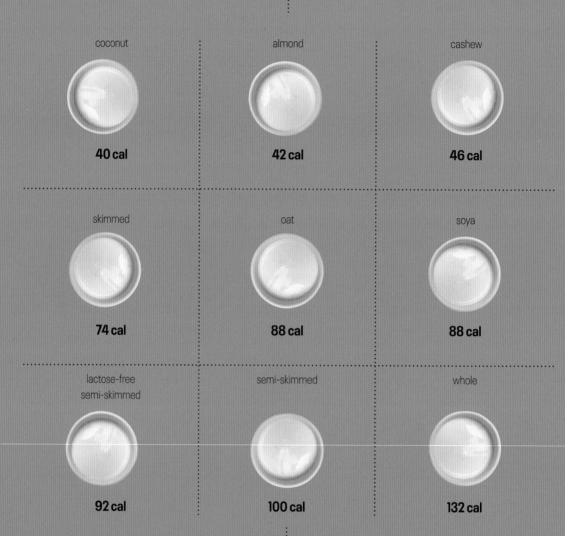

coconut	almond	cashew
40 cal	**42 cal**	**46 cal**

skimmed	oat	soya
74 cal	**88 cal**	**88 cal**

lactose-free semi-skimmed	semi-skimmed	whole
92 cal	**100 cal**	**132 cal**

Calories from milk – whether added to your cereal, tea or coffee – all add up too. There are some alternatives if you want to reduce your calories from milk, including non-dairy choices. However, despite the negative press it has received of late, dairy milk is an excellent source of nutrients.

BREAKFAST THAT APPARENTLY FILLS YOU UP

BREAKFAST THAT APPARENTLY MAKES YOU FAT

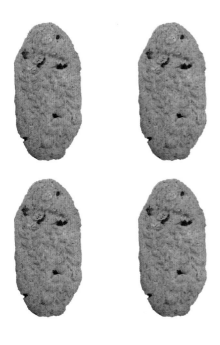

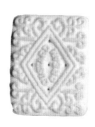
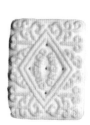
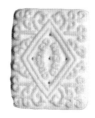
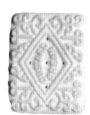

4 chocolate chip breakfast biscuits

280 cal

4 custard cream biscuits

232 cal

Breakfast biscuits are often marketed as 'healthy', specifically designed to keep you full for hours and fuel your entire morning. The reality is that a few biscuits, including breakfast varieties, are unlikely to fill you up. Eating your favourite biscuit could result in the same calorie consumption, or less, than a breakfast biscuit (and perhaps you'd enjoy it more). Choosing a breakfast that actually fills you up, and fits your calorie target, is the best option.

LOW-CALORIE FRY-UP

You can eat a fry-up if that is what you enjoy. Calorie savings can be made easily enough: use a non-stick pan and/or low-calorie cooking spray instead of oils or butter; use chicken sausages instead of pork or beef sausages; and bacon medallions instead of back or streaky bacon. Fry-ups also offer an excellent opportunity to include micronutrients too.

331 cal
31g protein

2 chicken sausages

3 bacon medallions

30g sliced mushrooms

10 sprays low-calorie oil

1 halved large tomato

1 medium egg

Preheat the oven to 200°C. Cook the chicken sausages on a roasting tray for 15 minutes (they need a head start).

Spray a large frying pan with low-calorie cooking oil, bring to a medium heat and add the sausages, bacon medallions, sliced mushrooms and a halved large tomato. Cook everything, for 10 minutes, turning half-way through, or until the bacon is nearly done.

Make space in the pan and add 1 medium egg. Cook everything for a further 3–5 minutes, or until the egg is done to your liking. Serve up!

COFFEE

medium
Americano

2 cal

medium
cappuccino

90 cal

medium
latte

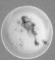

103 cal

medium
mocha

237 cal

medium
caramel latte

257 cal

large
Americano

3 cal

large
cappuccino

119 cal

large latte

141 cal

large mocha

353 cal

large
caramel latte

346 cal

If you like to drink coffee with breakfast, consider the calories and make sure your brew is not taking you over your calorie target. Can you switch your coffee preference – make it smaller, have it with less or a lighter milk, don't have a croissant as well...?

If you are not a fan of Americano, which has almost no calories, non-dairy milk alternatives are worth considering (see page 98) for their lower caloric content and some, such as almond or cashew nut, can enhance the flavour of the coffee.

HIGH-PROTEIN BREAKFAST IDEAS

Eating protein at breakfast will help you feel fuller for longer. Many brands are aware that health-conscious consumers seek protein. Beyond the marketing, a lot of manufactured breakfast products don't contain much protein and have a high caloric value. Read the label to see if the protein content in the product is a big enough helping to satisfy your needs and that the calories are within your target.

Ideally, make your own breakfast: it doesn't need to take long...

Berry & peanut butter porridge

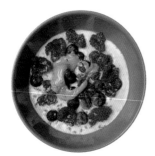

560 cal

43g protein

Add 50g of **oats** and 250ml of **semi-skimmed milk** to a microwaveable bowl. Microwave for 2–3 minutes until the oats begin to bubble. Remove from the microwave, mix in 30g of **whey powder**, a handful of **blueberries** and **raspberries**, 15g of **peanut butter**, 15g of **linseed**.

Chocolate & blackberry porridge

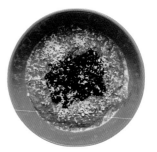

556 cal

42g protein

Add 50g of **oats** and 250ml of **semi-skimmed milk** to a microwaveable bowl. Microwave for 2–3 minutes until the oats begin to bubble. Remove from the microwave, mix in 30g of **chocolate whey powder**, 5 **blackberries** and 5g of **desiccated coconut**.

Jam pancakes

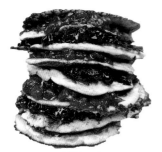

585 cal

35g protein

In a large mixing bowl, mix together 30g of **vanilla whey powder**, 1 **medium egg**, 50g of **0% Greek yogurt**. Melt 10g of **butter** in a large frying pan over a high heat. Ladle spoonfuls of batter into the pan to make as many pancakes as possible. Cook for 30–90 seconds on each side or until golden. Stack the pancakes on a plate, crushing **raspberries** and **blackberries** in between them to make a 'jam'. Pour over 20ml of **maple syrup**.

Chocolate protein pancakes

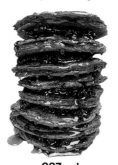

637 cal

39g protein

In a large mixing bowl, mix together 30g of **chocolate whey powder**, 1 **medium egg**, 1 **medium banana**, 50g of **0% Greek yogurt**. Melt 10g of **butter** in a large frying pan over a high heat. Ladle spoonfuls of batter into the pan to make as many pancakes as possible. Cook for 30–90 seconds on each side. Stack the pancakes on a plate, crushing **blackberries** in between them to make a 'jam'. Pour over 20ml of **maple syrup**.

Bacon & egg bagel

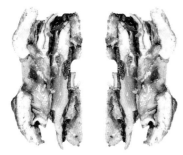

421 cal

40g protein

Heat 5ml of **olive oil** in a large frying pan over a medium heat. Add 4 **bacon medallions** and 2 **medium eggs** and cook for 7–10 minutes. Slice 1 **Bagel Thin** (widely available) and lightly toast. Sandwich with the bacon, eggs, 5ml of **tomato ketchup** and a small handful of **spinach**.

Yogurt & fruit protein bowl

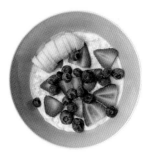

437 cal

48g protein

Add 200g of **0% fat Greek yogurt**, 25g of **oats** and 30g of **vanilla whey protein** to a bowl and mix. Then slice ½ **banana**, 3 medium **strawberries** and 30g of **blueberries** and add to the bowl.

FRENCH TOAST IDEAS

Introducing plenty of variety into your main meals, including breakfast, is not essential, but it may make long-term enjoyment of your overall diet more likely. Taking the basic recipe for French toast (bread dipped in egg), here are some simple ideas that will allow you to indulge your sweet or savoury tastes, depending on your preference. These will take you no more than about five minutes to prepare, and are a great way to start the day with some satisfying protein.

Basic French toast

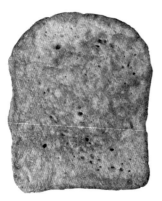

240 cal

10g protein

Heat 10ml of **olive oil** in a large frying pan. In a shallow bowl, whisk 1 **medium egg** then dip in 2 x 40g **slices of bread** until covered in the egg mixture. Add both slices to the hot pan and cook for 2 minutes on each side.

Smoked salmon with rocket & dill

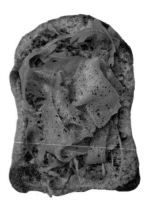

331 cal

22g protein

Top the cooked French toast with 50g of **smoked salmon**, a handful of **fresh rocket**, a sprinkling of **dried dill** and some **black pepper**.

Chorizo, spinach & cherry tomato

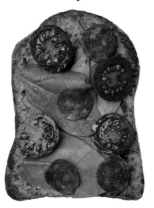

295 cal

13g protein

Top the cooked French toast with 10g of sliced **chorizo**, 2 sliced **cherry tomatoes** and a handful of **spinach leaves**.

Almond, chocolate dust & honey

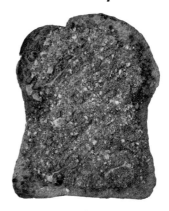

346 cal

12g protein

Blend together 15g of **milk chocolate** and 5 **almonds** to a powder. Spread evenly over the cooked French toast.

Strawberry & Greek yogurt

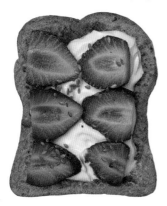

283 cal

16g protein

Top the cooked French toast with 50g of **0% fat Greek yogurt** and 3 sliced **strawberries**.

Nutella & raspberry

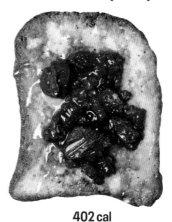

402 cal

11g protein

Top the cooked French toast with 1 tablespoon/ 15g of **Nutella**, 25g crushed **raspberries** and 10ml of **maple syrup**.

PIMP YOUR EGGS

Despite the largely media-driven concern over many years that eggs were detrimental to health because of their cholesterol content, recent evidence concludes that dietary cholesterol does not necessarily influence blood cholesterol (especially problematic LDL cholesterol). In the latest research, daily moderate consumption of eggs was shown to result in no increased risk of heart disease, or any other adverse health outcomes. In fact, across many studies, health markers improved. Eggs are a great source of high-quality protein, along with vitamins, minerals and iron, and a medium egg contains only 65 calories.

Basic omelette

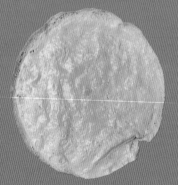

270 cal

Heat 10ml of mild **olive oil** in a medium pan. Whisk 3 **medium eggs** then add to the hot pan. Stir the mixture with a spatula as it cooks, for about 2 minutes.

Parma ham & mushroom omelette

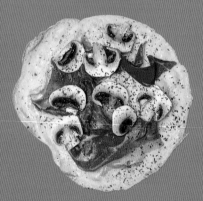

310 cal

Follow the basic omelette recipe then top with 2 slices of **Parma ham**, 2 chopped **mushrooms** and **black pepper**. Cook for a further 3 minutes and serve.

Chorizo & goat's cheese omelette

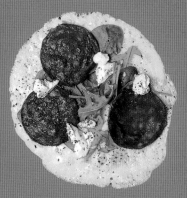

405 cal

Follow the basic omelette recipe then add 10g of sliced **chorizo**, 20g of **goat's cheese**, a handful of **rocket** and **spinach** and some **black pepper**. Cook for a further 3 minutes and serve.

Veggie omelette

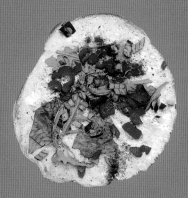

286 cal

Follow the basic omelette recipe then add ¼ chopped **red pepper**, ½ chopped **red onion**, a handful of **rocket** and 1 teaspoon of **paprika**. Cook for a further 3 minutes and serve.

Simple scrambled eggs on toast

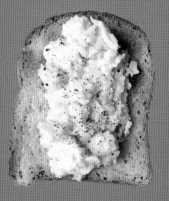

225 cal

Whisk 2 **medium eggs** and add to a small, non-stick pan over a low heat. Cook for 4–6 minutes, stirring the mixture with a spoon or spatula. Toast a 40g slice of **bread** and top with the scrambled eggs, **salt** and **black pepper**.

Poached egg & avocado on toast

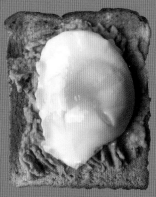

243 cal

Bring a saucepan of water to a simmer (small bubbles) and crack in 1 **medium egg**. Poach for 3–5 minutes or until set. Mash ¼ of a medium **avocado**. Toast a 40g slice of **bread**. Spread the toast with avocado and top with the poached egg.

NAVIGATING
LUNCH
& DINNER

As the foods we eat for lunch and dinner are often similar, I've grouped these meal ideas together. However, you should eat according to your schedule – if the traditional three meals a day fits your lifestyle, then great. That said, rigidily sticking to eating three meals a day isn't the only way to lose weight.

The number of meals you eat each day should align with your preferences. For some people, four–six smaller meals may suit their day whereas, for others, two larger meals may be better.

The bottom line is: your total calorie intake is what matters, not the number of meals you choose to eat or how regularly they are consumed. There is no conclusive evidence, across the body of scientific research available, to prove that a specific number of meals is best for fat loss.

What is best for fat loss is a calorie deficit. And what has also been shown to help adherence to a calorie deficit is consuming protein. Ensure that you have a meaningful portion of protein (25–50g) in most meals, if possible.

Lunch can be the most problematic meal of the day, often eaten and purchased outside the sphere of your control. It's far better to make your own lunches – and dinners – from scratch at home. While a typical shop-bought sandwich, ready meal, chocolate bar or packet of crisps may be your preference (and on point with societal norms), the key to achieving your goals is to be in control of what you eat most of the time.

If your regular lunch choice fits within your daily or weekly calorie target, leaves you with sufficient calories to enjoy at other times during the day, and keeps you feeling full, then you don't need to alter your habits. However, if it doesn't deliver on all three counts, then you need to make adjustments, either to other meals you eat during the day, or make changes to your usual preferred lunch choice.

'I DON'T HAVE TIME TO COOK DINNER'

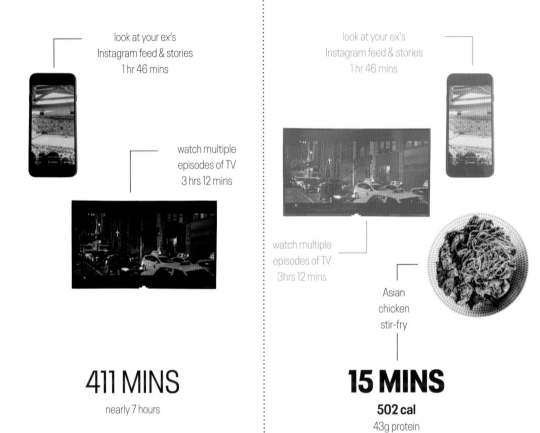

look at your ex's
Instagram feed & stories
1 hr 46 mins

look at your ex's
Instagram feed & stories
1 hr 46 mins

watch multiple
episodes of TV
3 hrs 12 mins

watch multiple
episodes of TV
3hrs 12 mins

Asian
chicken
stir-fry

411 MINS
nearly 7 hours

15 MINS
502 cal
43g protein

Time is what we make of it. Just 15 minutes spent cooking is more meaningful than hours of despairing because of zero progress.

You CAN find time to prepare meals each day, and in most cases, at no cost to your Instagram scrolling, Netflix indulging or WhatsApp marathons.

You just need to choose to dedicate a small segment of your life to it.

'DON'T EAT CARBS
AFTER 6PM'

5.59PM   **6.01PM**

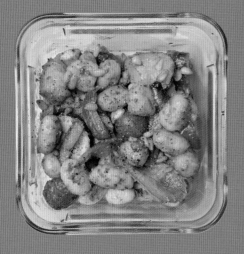

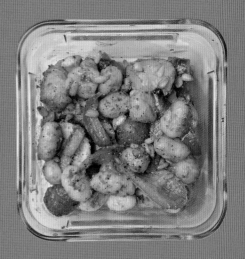

432 calorie meal   **432 calorie meal**
57g carbs   57g carbs

The old adage 'don't eat carbs after 6pm' is, in fact, unproven. The majority of research shows that it doesn't matter when we eat carbs (or any food), but it does matter how many calories we consume.

If you like eating early, do that. If you like eating later, you can do that too.

NOT WORTH TRACKING
per week

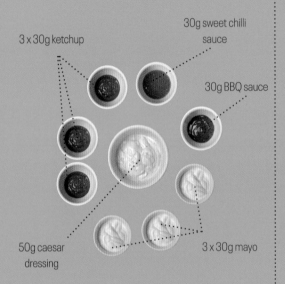

3 x 30g ketchup

30g sweet chilli sauce

30g BBQ sauce

50g caesar dressing

3 x 30g mayo

1,135 cal

I'VE BLOWN MY DIET
per week

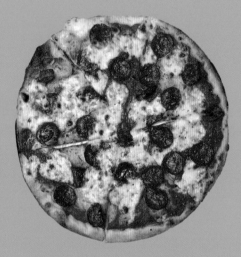

1 x Domino's small Italian crust pepperoni pizza

1,085 cal

It is wise to become consistently aware of your eating behaviours. Get rid of any assumptions – such as, condiments don't make much of a difference – and replace them with facts. For example, this selection of generous, yet normalized, servings of sauces adds up to 1,135 calories. You might assume that each portion of sauce is small enough to omit from your calorie counting but, while individually small, over time (say a week), they add up to be large.

You might assume that you can eat all these condiments without impacting on your fat loss but that a high-calorie pizza would be a disaster. But since this pizza has fewer calories than all the sauces, you could lose all the sauces and eat the pizza instead.

Be aware of your eating patterns and how they may be impacting on your progress. But also remember that all food is allowed.

FISH & SEAFOOD

(per 100g)

prawns	crayfish	mussels	squid	lobster
62 cal	**75 cal**	**83 cal**	**84 cal**	**95 cal**
14g protein	17g protein	17g protein	16g protein	20g protein

cod	tuna	seabass	mackerel	salmon
81 cal	**124 cal**	**157 cal**	**208 cal**	**208 cal**
18g protein	28g protein	19g protein	25g protein	25g protein

Fish and seafood offer us a dense source of protein. As with meat, some sources can contain more fat than others, but – unlike the saturated fat in meat – the fat in oily fish, such as salmon and mackerel, which are highest in calories, contains omega-3 fatty acids, which have been shown to benefit heart health. This may be a consideration when planning your meat to fish ratio across meals.

MEAT

(per 100g)

kangaroo	chicken breast	turkey breast mince	5% fat beef mince	ham
100 cal	**105 cal**	**112 cal**	**125 cal**	**145 cal**
24g protein	25g protein	25g protein	21g protein	21g protein
bacon	fillet steak	venison	veal	bison
180 cal	**155 cal**	**160 cal**	**170 cal**	**170 cal**
16g protein	21g protein	30g protein	23g protein	23g protein
lamb cutlet	duck	chicken drumstick	pork chop	rib-eye
175 cal	**175 cal**	**235 cal**	**270 cal**	**255 cal**
30g protein	28g protein	19g protein	18g protein	19g protein

Animal meat offers a dense source of protein, which helps us feel full and maintains our muscle mass. As you can see, most meat sources are similar in protein value, whereas red meat tends to be more calorie dense – this is because of its fat content. Poultry tends to be lower in calories simply because it contains less fat. There are no carbohydrates in fresh meat or poultry.

CALORIE-SAVING MEAT SWAPS

200g chicken thighs	200g rib-eye steak	2 back bacon rashers (60g)	200g beef mince	2 pork sausages (120g)

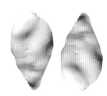 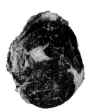 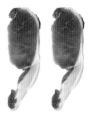 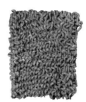

322 cal	**510 cal**	**108 cal**	**503 cal**	**330 cal**
36g protein	38g protein	10g protein	36g protein	24g protein

200g chicken breasts	200g fillet steak	2 back bacon medallions (60g)	200g turkey breast mince	2 chicken sausages (120g)

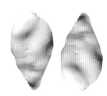 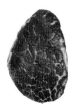 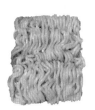 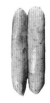

210 cal	**312 cal**	**45 cal**	**227 cal**	**163 cal**
48g protein	42g protein	9g protein	50g protein	25g protein

All of the choices on the top row can be enjoyed as part of a balanced, protein-rich diet. Those on the bottom row offer a similar tasting option with fewer calories, less fat and more protein, with the exception of the bacon medallions.

If the top row was swapped for the bottom row over the course of five meals, you would save 649 calories with no drastic alteration to your diet. Processed meat can be eaten, but recent evidence, recommends we limit consumption to below 50g a day.

VEGETABLES
(per 100g)

For some, the primary use of vegetables is to initiate sexually heightened exchanges on a smartphone. But, in real life, vegetables serve as an outstanding source of energy because they contain essential vitamins and minerals, fibre and body-hydrating water. A diet rich in a variety of vegetables undoubtedly supports our overall health. It can also help facilitate a calorie deficit because many vegetables are low in calories and high in fibre, which fills us up.

mushrooms

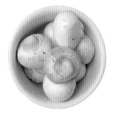

8 cal

courgette

20 cal

aubergine

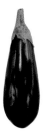

20 cal

asparagus

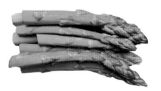

28 cal

spinach

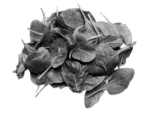

29 cal

green beans

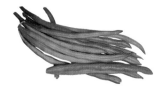

31 cal

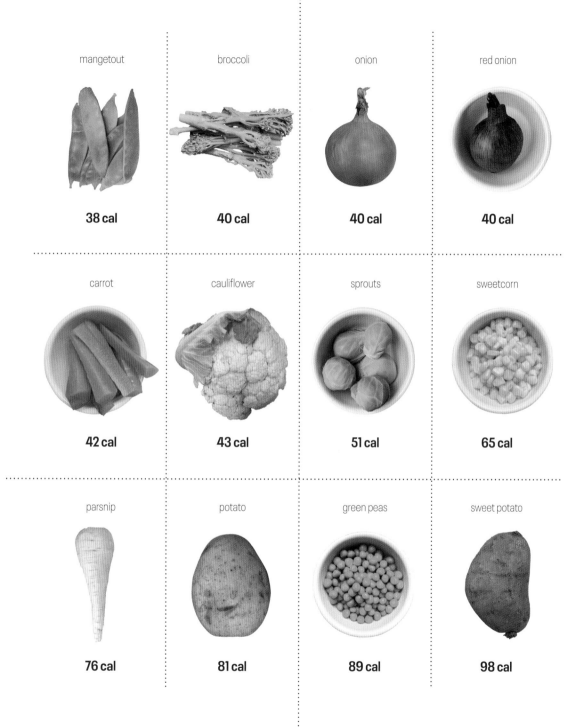

mangetout	broccoli	onion	red onion
38 cal	**40 cal**	**40 cal**	**40 cal**
carrot	cauliflower	sprouts	sweetcorn
42 cal	**43 cal**	**51 cal**	**65 cal**
parsnip	potato	green peas	sweet potato
76 cal	**81 cal**	**89 cal**	**98 cal**

BAGEL IDEAS

A typical plain bagel, weighing 105g, is about 240 calories. Here are fresh ideas, old favourites and new combos to try. Some lend themselves to a lunch on the go and others make for a tasty midday meal for days when you're at home. If you want to reduce calories further, you can swap a regular bagel for a bagel thin, which contains around 110 calories. But these ideas are all based on the traditional 240-calorie bagel.

Note: If you don't want to toast the bagels, don't toast them.

Fried egg & fresh watercress

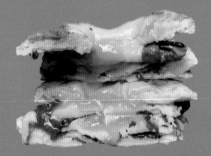

481 cal
26g protein

Heat 5ml of **olive oil** in a frying pan, add a handful of **watercress** and crack in 3 **medium eggs**. Fry for 4–6 minutes until the watercress is wilted and the eggs are cooked how you like them. Split and toast 1 bagel, top with the fried eggs and watercress, and season with **salt and pepper**.

Bacon & mozzarella

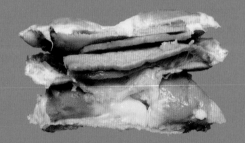

534 cal
34g protein

Split and toast 1 bagel. Grill 3 rashers of **bacon** for 5 minutes on each side or until crisp. Top the bagel with the bacon and 20g of **light mozzarella**. Put the loaded bagel back under the grill for 3 minutes or until the mozzarella is melted.

Smoked salmon & feta bagel

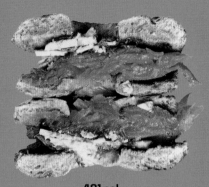

481 cal
34g protein

Split and toast 1 **bagel** then top with 100g of **smoked salmon**, 25g of **feta cheese** and 1 teaspoon of fresh or dried chopped **dill**.

Chicken, chorizo & rocket

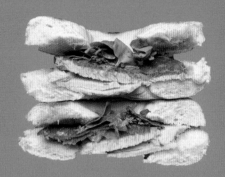

517 cal
43g protein

Split and toast 1 bagel then spread with 10g of **light mayonnaise**, 100g of cooked, sliced **chicken breast**, 10g of **chorizo** slices and some **rocket**.

Houmous & roasted red pepper

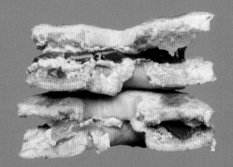

445 cal
12g protein

Split and toast 1 bagel then spread with 50g **houmous** and top with ½ chopped **red pepper**.

Chicken & avocado

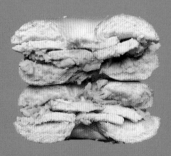

575 cal
36g protein

Split and toast 1 bagel. Mash ½ medium **avocado** and spread over one half of the bagel then top with 100g of cooked, sliced **chicken breast** and season with **salt and pepper**.

CHICKEN SANDWICH

Here, the pimped version has more calories, but eating its extra ingredients will also bring you greater enjoyment. A diet of monotonous, bland food will not help you enjoy losing weight or cultivate a long-term calorie deficit. Choose tasty food that adds textures and flavours while keeping you within your calorie target. Do not try to cut your calories too quickly or in extreme ways.

2 x 40g slices wholemeal bread
160 cal

75g cooked chicken breast
180 cal

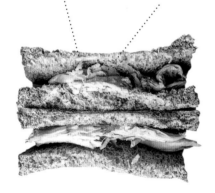

30g goat's cheese
80 cal

2 x 40g slices wholemeal bread
160 cal

10g chilli pesto
30 cal

2 sliced cherry tomatoes
3 cal

75g cooked chicken breast
180 cal

3 slices cucumber
3 cal

few spinach leaves
2 cal

PLAIN
340 cal
(*tastes OK)

PIMPED
458 cal
(*more nutrients & party in your mouth)

GREEK-STYLE NACHO SALAD

540 cal
15g protein

2 flatbreads
221 cal

3 medium tomatoes
66 cal

½ small avocado
88 cal

30g feta cheese
75 cal

small handful of
chives & coriander
0 cal

handful of spinach,
juice of 1 lime,
10ml olive oil,
salt & pepper
90 cal

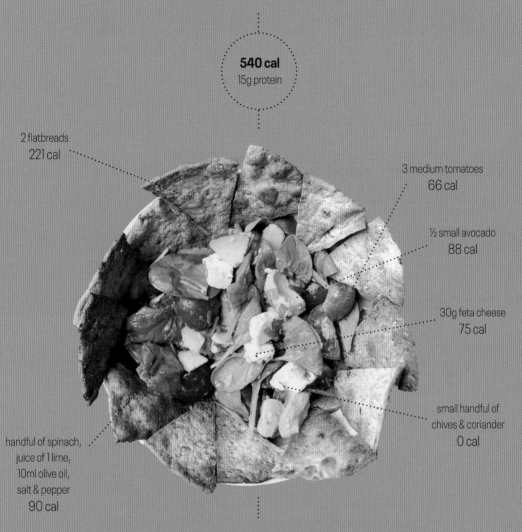

Preheat the oven to 200°C. Cut the flatbreads into triangles and lay on a foil-lined baking tray then bake in the oven for 5 minutes until golden and crispy.

Chop the tomatoes, avocado, feta cheese, chives and coriander. Mix together with the spinach, the juice of 1 lime, 10ml of olive oil, salt and pepper. Toss together. Eat with your homemade nachos.

BAKED SEABASS

429 cal
43g protein

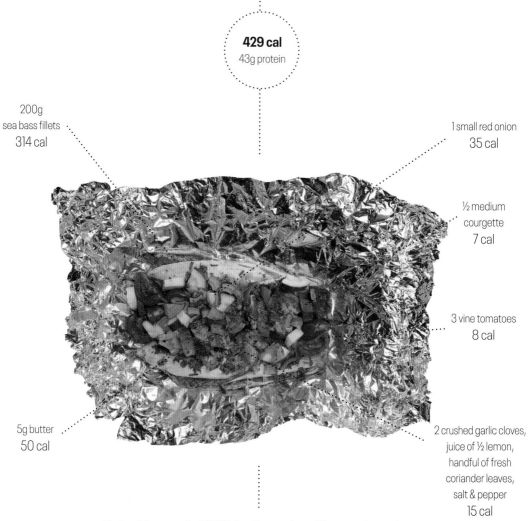

200g
sea bass fillets
314 cal

1 small red onion
35 cal

½ medium
courgette
7 cal

3 vine tomatoes
8 cal

5g butter
50 cal

2 crushed garlic cloves,
juice of ½ lemon,
handful of fresh
coriander leaves,
salt & pepper
15 cal

Preheat the oven to 200°C. Lay the sea bass fillets on a large sheet of foil on a baking tray. Dot the butter over each fillet. Finely chop the onion and courgette, slice or quarter the tomatoes and arrange on top of the fish. Crush the garlic cloves over the veg and squeeze over the lemon juice. Finish with the fresh coriander leaves and season with salt and pepper.

Fold the foil sheet loosely around the fish and seal to make a parcel. Cook in the hot oven for 20 minutes, unfold the foil and eat.

SALMON TAGLIATELLE

562 cal
38g protein

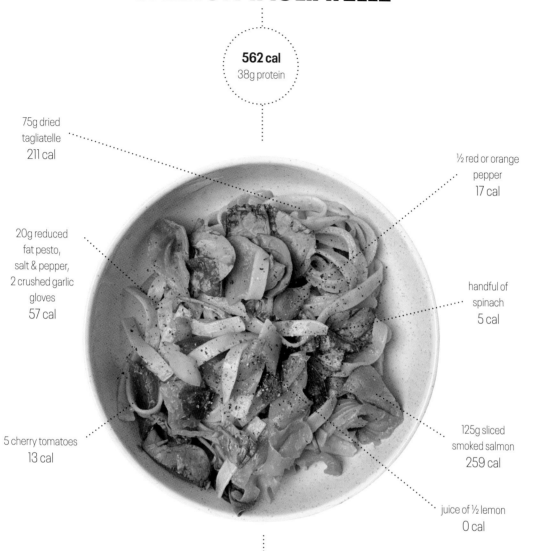

75g dried
tagliatelle
211 cal

½ red or orange
pepper
17 cal

20g reduced
fat pesto,
salt & pepper,
2 crushed garlic
gloves
57 cal

handful of
spinach
5 cal

5 cherry tomatoes
13 cal

125g sliced
smoked salmon
259 cal

juice of ½ lemon
0 cal

Bring a large pan of water to the boil, drop in the dried tagliatelle
and cook for 6–8 minutes or follow the packet instructions. Drain
and mix with the red pesto, some salt and pepper and 2 crushed
garlic cloves. Add the sliced or chopped cherry tomatoes, chopped
pepper, a handful of spinach and the smoked salmon. Squeeze over
the lemon juice and mix everything together before serving. Ideal
for dinner, great to make for a work lunch the next day too!

DOUBLE CHICKEN CHEESE BURGER

653 cal
53g protein

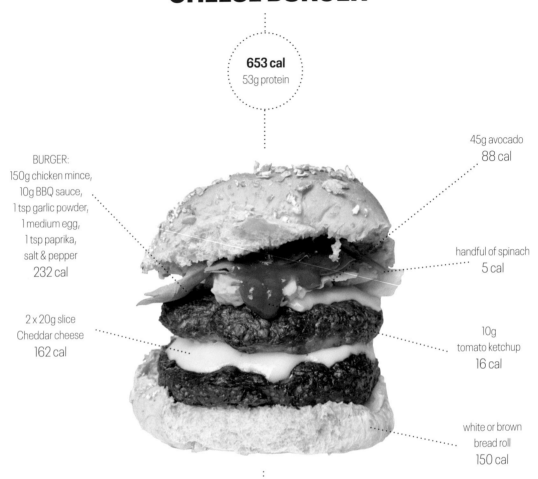

BURGER:
150g chicken mince,
10g BBQ sauce,
1 tsp garlic powder,
1 medium egg,
1 tsp paprika,
salt & pepper
232 cal

45g avocado
88 cal

handful of spinach
5 cal

2 x 20g slice
Cheddar cheese
162 cal

10g
tomato ketchup
16 cal

white or brown
bread roll
150 cal

Preheat the oven to 200°C. In a large bowl, mix 150g of chicken mince, 10g of BBQ sauce, 1 teaspoon of garlic powder, 1 medium egg, 1 teaspoon of paprika and some salt and pepper. Form into 2 balls then press down to shape into two burgers. Transfer to a foil-lined baking tray and cook for 30 minutes in the hot oven. For the last 5 minutes of cooking, put a 20g slice of Cheddar cheese on top of each burger to melt. Split the bread roll and mash avocado. Layer the cheese burgers inside the roll with mashed avocado, spinach and tomato ketchup.

MEXICAN CHICKEN MEAL

503 cal
52g protein

MARINADE:
+
½ red pepper,
½ orange pepper
33 cal
+
10ml olive oil
80 cal
+
1 tsp chilli powder,
1 tbsp garlic powder,
1 tsp ground cumin,
1 tbsp dried oregano,
1 tbsp dried parsley,
50ml water
tasty AF

200g chicken breast
210 cal

50g dried egg
noodles
180 cal

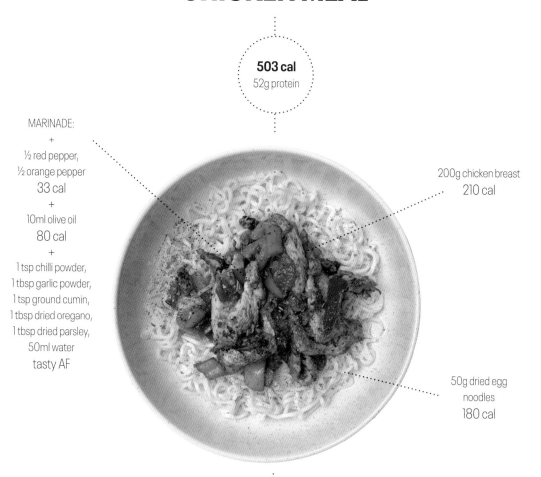

In a large bowl, mix together all the ingredients for the marinade.

Roughly chop 200g chicken breast and add to the bowl with the marinade mix. Stir to coat, then refrigerate for 1 hour. After 1 hour, heat a frying pan and add the marinated chicken. Cook for 10–15 minutes or until cooked through. Bring a saucepan of water to the boil, add the dried egg noodles and cook for 5–8 minutes or follow the packet instructions. Drain, then tip the noodles onto a plate and top with the cooked chicken.

BANGERS & MASH

TASTY

STILL TASTY

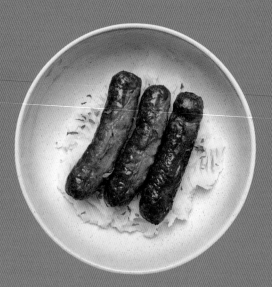

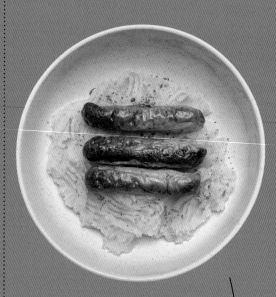

807 cal
48g protein

361 cal
43g protein

Preheat the oven to 200°C. Put 3 **chicken sausages** on a foil-lined baking tray and cook in the hot oven for about 35 minutes or until piping hot and nicely browned. Meanwhile, bring a saucepan of water to the boil then add 75g of chopped **carrot**, 75g of chopped **swede**, 1 crushed **garlic clove** and 75g of chopped **parsnip**. Cook for 10 minutes until tender. Drain then mash the vegetables with 10 sprays of **low-calorie olive oil**, 100g of **0% fat Greek yogurt**, **salt** and **pepper**. Serve with the sausages on top.

SPAGHETTI BOLOGNESE

TASTY

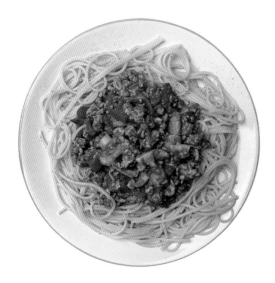

875 cal

55g protein

STILL TASTY

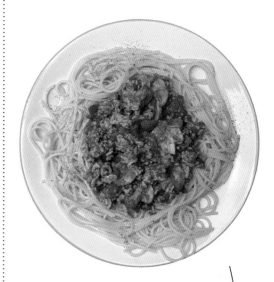

587 cal

58g protein

Heat 5 sprays of l**ow-calorie oil** in a frying pan over a medium heat then add 200g of **5%-fat beef mince**. Cook for 5 minutes, stirring, until browned all over. Add 1 chopped **red pepper**, 1 chopped **red onion**, 100g of **mushrooms** and 200ml of **passata**. Reduce the heat and cook for 10 minutes. Meanwhile, bring a saucepan of water to the boil and add 50g of dried s**paghetti**. Cook for 6–8 minutes or follow the packet instructions. Drain the pasta, serve topped with the bolognese sauce and sprinkled with **dried coriander**, and **salt** and **pepper**.

PAN-FRIED GNOCCHI

TASTY

STILL TASTY

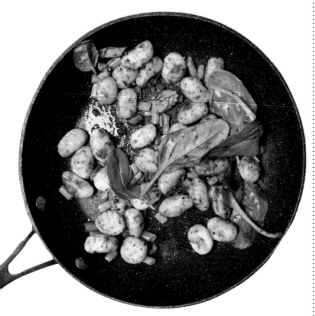

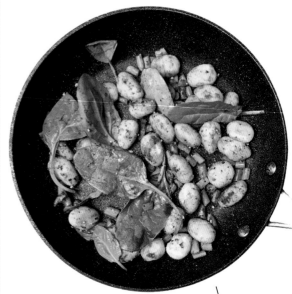

645 cal
16g protein

551 cal
16g protein

Heat 10 sprays of **low-calorie oil** in a frying pan over a medium heat. Add 250g of **gnocchi** to the pan and cook for 5 minutes, then add 30g of chopped **green beans**, 1 tablespoon of **light red pesto**, 1 teaspoon of **paprika** and a handful of **spinach**. Cook over a low heat for a further 5 minutes, season with **salt** and **pepper**, then eat.

CHICKEN STIR-FRY

TASTY

STILL TASTY

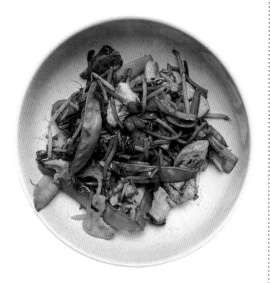

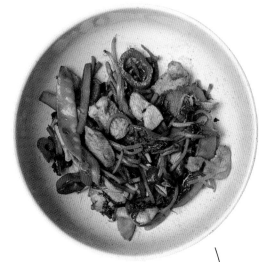

388 cal

41g protein

316 cal

41g protein

Heat 10 sprays of **low-calorie oil** in a frying pan over a medium heat, then add 150g of chopped **chicken breast** and cook, stirring, for 5 minutes. Add 20ml of **soy sauce**, 50g of **mangetout**, 50g of **bean sprouts**, ½ chopped **red pepper**, a handful of **spinach** and ½ **chopped onion**. Stir-fry everything for 6–8 minutes, then eat.

CHILLI CON CARNE

TASTY

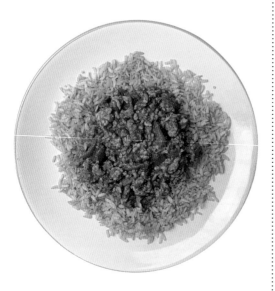

876 cal

56g protein

STILL TASTY

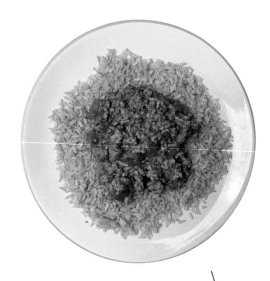

588 cal

56g protein

Heat 10 sprays of **low-calorie oil** in a frying pan over a medium heat. Add 200g of **5%-fat beef mince** and cook for 5 minutes or until browned. Add 1 tablespoon ground **cumin**, 200ml **passata**, ½ a standard (400g) can of **mixed beans**, 1 chopped **onion** and ½ red **pepper** and simmer for 10 minutes on low heat. Serve with 125g cooked **brown or white rice** and some sliced **red chilli**, season with **salt** and **pepper**.

FISH 'N' CHIPS

TASTY

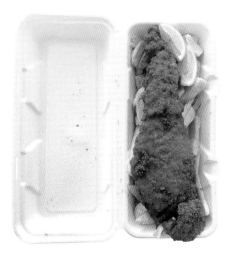

STILL TASTY

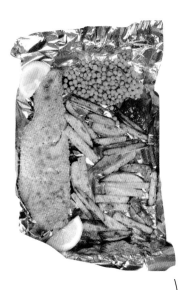

946 cal
45g protein

588 cal
52g protein

Preheat the oven to 200°C. Whisk 1 **medium egg** in a large bowl. Put 50g **breadcrumbs** (bought or homemade) in another bowl. Dip a 150g fresh **cod fillet** first in the egg, making sure it is fully coated, then in the breadcrumbs to cover the fish evenly. Slice 200g **potatoes** into chips and add to a mixing bowl with 5ml of **olive oil**, a pinch of salt, 1 teaspoon of **garlic powde**r and 1 teaspoon of dried **mixed herbs**. Mix with your hands to coat the potatoes fully. Put the fish and potato chips on a non-stick or foil-lined baking tray in a single layer and cook in the hot oven for 30–35 minutes. Five minutes before the end of the cooking, bring a saucepan of water to the boil and cook 50g of fresh or frozen **peas**. Drain the peas and serve everything with 10g **tomato ketchup** and **lemon wedges**.

PIRI PIRI CHICKEN NOODLES

497 cal
41g protein

MARINADE:
1 garlic clove,
10ml vinegar,
½ red chilli,
1 tsp smoked paprika,
juice of ½ lime,
5ml olive oil
55 cal

50g dried rice noodles
181 cal

½ red chilli,
salt & pepper
5 cal

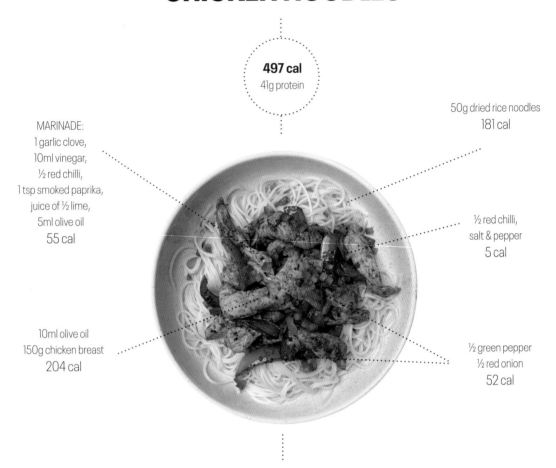

10ml olive oil
150g chicken breast
204 cal

½ green pepper
½ red onion
52 cal

Mix together all the ingredients for the marinade – I use a nutribullet. Heat the olive oil in a frying pan over a high heat, then add the roughly chopped chicken breast. Cook the chicken for 2 minutes on each side, or until browned all over, then reduce the heat to low and cook for 10 minutes or until cooked through. Bring a saucepan of water to the boil and cook the rice noodles for 3–5 minutes or follow the packet instructions. Chop the green pepper and red onion then mix them and the cooked chicken and the peri peri marinade. Drain the noodles and plate up with the peri peri chicken, peppers and onion. Top with the finely chopped red chilli and season with salt and black pepper.

COURGETTE & SWEETCORN FRITTERS

478 cal
32g protein

FRITTERS:
1 medium egg
30g self-raising flour
80g sweetcorn
½ courgette, grated
1 tsp paprika
salt & pepper
268 cal

3 medium eggs
195 cal

handful of spinach
5 cal

10 sprays of low-calorie oil
10 cal

1 tsp sriracha
0 cal

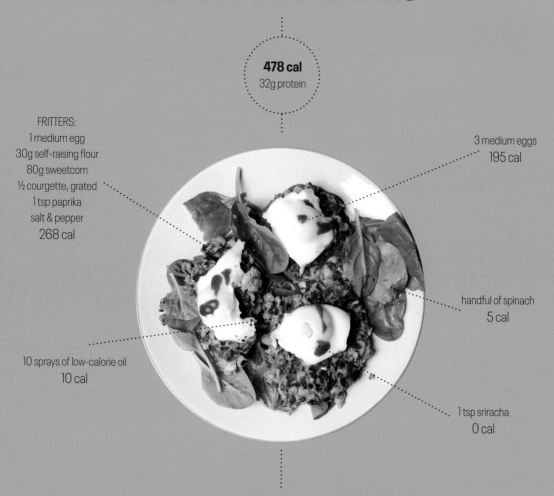

For the fritters, mix together the egg, flour, sweetcorn, grated courgette, paprika, salt and pepper. Form 3 evenly sized balls from the mixture. Heat 10 sprays of low-calorie oil in a frying pan over a medium heat. Add the balls to the hot pan and press down with a spoon or your hand to form 3cm-thick fritters in the pan. Cook for 5–7 minutes on each side. Bring a saucepan of water to a simmer and poach 3 medium eggs for 3–5 minutes or until cooked how you like them. Serve the poached eggs on top of the fritters and serve with a handful of spinach leaves and drizzle with sriracha.

TURKEY CHORIZO RAGU

581 cal
48g protein

10ml olive oil
80 cal

50g dried
penne pasta
128 cal

150g turkey mince
168 cal

15g chorizo
slices
70 cal

1 tsp ground turmeric,
1 tsp garlic powder,
1 tsp dried oregano,
20g red pesto,
½ red pepper
92 cal

10g grated
Parmesan cheese
43 cal

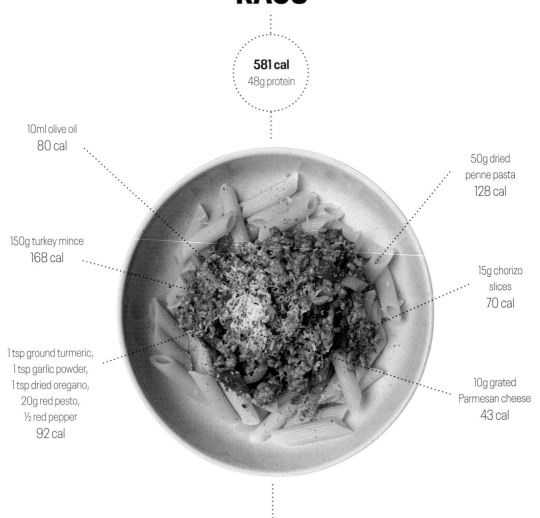

Heat the olive oil in a frying pan over a high heat then add the turkey mince, the spices, dried oregano, regular red pesto and chopped red pepper. Cook for 10 minutes, stirring regularly. Bring a saucepan of water to the boil, add a pinch of salt and the penne. Cook the pasta for 5–7 minutes or follow the packet instructions. Drain. Add the chorizo slices to the turkey mince in the pan. Serve the penne topped with the ragu and sprinkled with Parmesan cheese.

QUORN RAGU

553 cal
34g protein

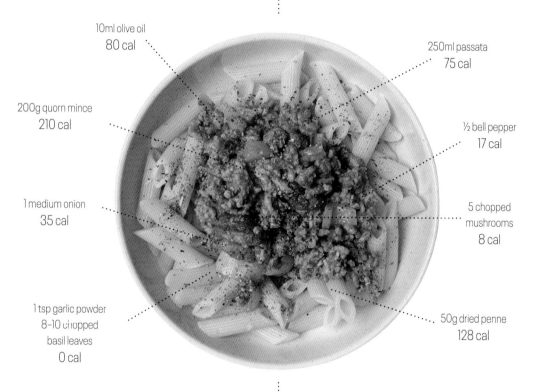

10ml olive oil
80 cal

250ml passata
75 cal

200g quorn mince
210 cal

½ bell pepper
17 cal

1 medium onion
35 cal

5 chopped
mushrooms
8 cal

1 tsp garlic powder
8-10 chopped
basil leaves
0 cal

50g dried penne
128 cal

Heat the olive oil in a frying pan before adding the quorn mince, chopped onion, garlic powder and chopped basil. Cook for 5 minutes before adding passata, chopped bell pepper, chopped mushrooms and chopped basil. Turn heat down and simmer for a further 10 minutes, stirring regularly. Meanwhile, bring water in a saucepan to boil and heat penne for 4-6 minutes until tender. Drain penne and serve with quorn ragu.

LOW-CALORIE PIZZA IDEAS

Tortillas make brilliant pizza bases and offer a quick solution for a midweek supper when time is short and you want to make a tasty meal fast. The toppings here include cooked white meat, such as chicken breast or turkey mince, and the more traditional cured meats, such as ham and salami. Soft goat's cheese and mozzarella are low-calorie alternatives to hard cheeses like Parmesan, while sliced vegetables, herbs and leaves add flavour, interest and colour. For all pizzas, preheat the oven to 200°C, then add the following toppings to a medium tortilla and cook for 8–10 minutes or until the cheese has melted.

Chicken & mozarella

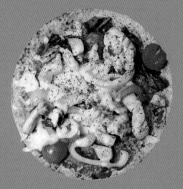

406 cal
32g protein

Top the tortilla with: 20g of **tomato purée**, 75g of cooked **chicken breast**, ½ chopped yellow **pepper**, 4 sliced **cherry tomatoes**, a handful of **spinach**, 25g of **low-fat mozzarella** and 1 teaspoon of **dried parsley**.

Ham & chorizo

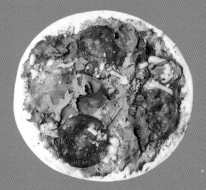

476 cal
27g protein

Top the tortilla with: 20g of **tomato purée**, 1 teaspoon of **dried parsley**, 15g of **chorizo** slices, 20g of sliced **ham**, a handful each of **spinach** and **rocket** and 50g of **low-fat mozzarella**.

Meat feast

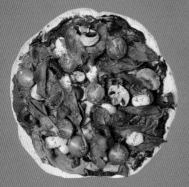

488 cal

28g protein

Top the tortilla with: 20g of **tomato purée**, 1 teaspoon of **garlic powder**, ¼ chopped **red pepper**, 2 sliced **mushrooms**, 4 sliced **cherry tomatoes**, 30g of **goat's cheese**, 3 slices of **Parma ham**, 10g of **salami**, and a handful of **spinach**.

Bolognese

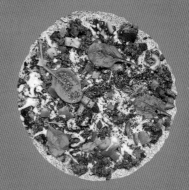

587 cal

38g protein

Top the tortilla with: 125g of **turkey ragu** (see page 134), 50g of **low-fat mozzarella**, ¼ chopped **green pepper** and a handful of **spinach**.

BBQ chicken & chorizo

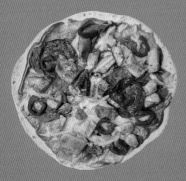

558 cal

44g protein

Top the tortilla with: 75g or cooked chicken breast, 10g of **BBQ sauce**, 50g of **low-fat mozzarella**, 2 slices of **chorizo**, a handful of **spinach**, ⅛ chopped **red pepper** and 1 teaspoon of dried **Italian herbs**.

Veggie

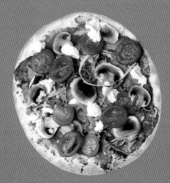

310 cal

11g protein

Top the tortilla with: 20g of **tomato purée**, 1 teaspoon of **paprika**, 30g of **goat's cheese**, a handful each of **spinach** and **rocket**, 2 sliced **mushrooms**, 3 sliced **cherry tomatoes** and 20g sliced **courgette**.

QUICK
CURRY IDEAS

Curries are often consumed on social occasions and whilst it is absolutely ok to eat them, most restaurants and takeaway curries are particularly calorie dense. If eaten regularly, thousands of calories in one sitting could affect your progress. If you enjoy going out for a curry and want to lose weight, it's wise to moderate consumption. Here are a few low-calorie curry recipes that can be made easily at home.

TAKEAWAY CURRY, RICE AND NAAN

onion bhajis

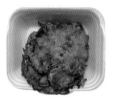

485 cal

aloo dum

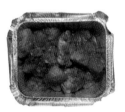

315 cal

naan

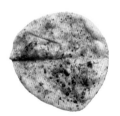

761 cal

pilau rice

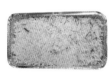

514 cal

chicken tikka masala

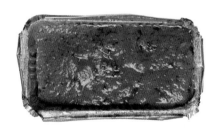

1,037 cal

3,112 cal

Thai green curry

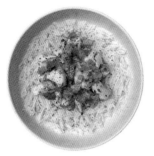

581 cal

Heat 10ml of **olive oil** in a frying pan, then add 150g of **chicken breast**, 100g of Thai green curry paste, a large handful of **fresh coriander**, 2 tablespoons of **0% fat Greek yogurt**, 1 chopped **green pepper** and ½ chopped **red onion**. Cook for 15 minutes. While the curry is cooking, heat up 125g cooked **basmati rice**. Serve.

Prawn & Sweet Potato Balti

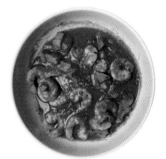

469 cal

Heat 10ml of **olive oil** in a frying pan, then add 150g of **cooked prawns**, 2 tablespoons of **Balti curry paste**, 1 teaspoon of ground **cumin** and 100g of **passata**. Cook for 15 minutes. While the curry is cooking, microwave 150g chopped **sweet potato** for 5–7 minutes or until tender. Serve.

Lamb masala tear-up naan

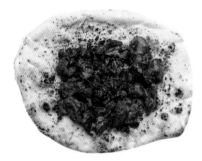

574 cal

Heat 10ml of **olive oil** in a frying pan, then add 200g of **diced lamb**, 3 tablespoons of **masala paste**, a handful of **spinach** and ½ chopped **red chilli**. Cook for 5 minutes. Place a 175g **garlic & coriander naan** under a hot grill for 2 minutes or until piping hot. Serve.

Chicken tikka masala

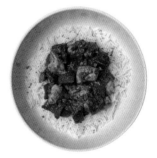

555 cal

Heat 10ml of **olive oil** in a frying pan, then add 150g of **chicken breast**, 2 tbsp of **masala paste**, 100g of **passata**, ½ **red onion**, 5 chopped **cherry tomatoes**, some **fresh basil** and ½ chopped **red pepper**. While the curry is cooking, heat up 125g cooked **basmati rice**. Serve.

STEAK & EGGS

606 cal
52g protein

MARINADE:
10ml olive oil,
1 tbsp paprika,
2 crushed garlic cloves,
salt
85 cal

150g sirloin steak
301 cal

100g sweet potato
98 cal

1 red onion,
½ red pepper
52 cal

1 medium egg
65 cal

handful of spinach
5 cal

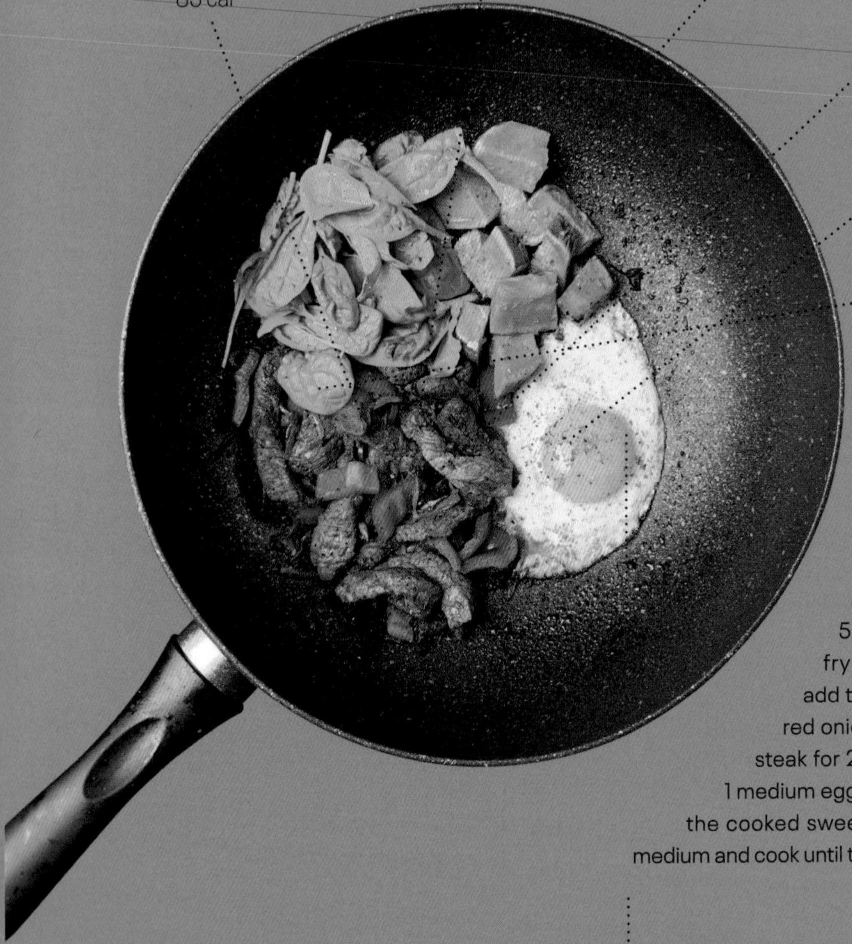

In a large bowl, mix the ingredients for the marinade. Slice up a 200g sirloin steak and coat with the marinade. Roughly chop the sweet potato and cook in the microwave for 5–7 minutes or until soft. Heat a frying pan over a high heat then add the marinated steak, 1 chopped red onion and ½ red pepper. Sear the steak for 2–4 minutes before cracking in 1 medium egg. Add a handful of spinach and the cooked sweet potato. Reduce the heat to medium and cook until the egg is how you like it. Eat.

PAPRIKA SALMON & WEDGES

541cal
33g protein

10ml olive oil
1 tsp paprika
1 tsp dried basil
pinch of salt
80 cal

200g
sweet potato
196 cal

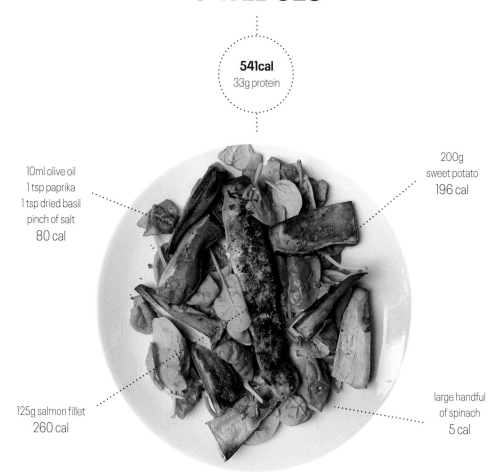

125g salmon fillet
260 cal

large handful
of spinach
5 cal

Preheat the oven to 220°C. Mix together the olive oil, paprika, dried basil and a pinch of salt in a small bowl, then rub over the salmon fillet. Slice the sweet potato into wedges and rub with any remaining salmon seasoning. Put the salmon and wedges on a non-stick or foil-lined baking tray and cook in the hot oven for 15 minutes. Serve the cooked salmon and wedges with a large handful of spinach.

CHICKEN SATAY

640 cal
57g protein

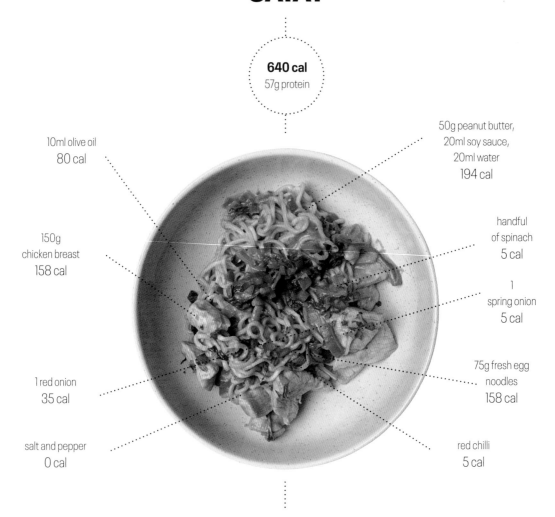

10ml olive oil
80 cal

50g peanut butter,
20ml soy sauce,
20ml water
194 cal

handful
of spinach
5 cal

150g
chicken breast
158 cal

1
spring onion
5 cal

1 red onion
35 cal

75g fresh egg
noodles
158 cal

salt and pepper
0 cal

red chilli
5 cal

Heat the olive oil in a frying pan, add the chopped chicken breast and chopped red onion and cook over a high heat for 5 minutes to brown the chicken. Reduce the heat to medium, add the peanut butter, soy sauce and water, stirring to coat the chicken. Add the spinach, and chopped spring onion. Simmer for 5 minutes or until the onion is soft and the chicken cooked through. Add the egg noodles and cook for a further 5 minutes before seasoning. Serve sprinkled with chopped red chilli.

PLANNING YOUR
SNACKS

A snack is simply an amount of food consumed between larger meals. It is not bad or something to feel guilty about.

Snacking between meals does not automatically mean you will become fat.

When you are hungry, it's usually a sign that you should eat.

If you are trying to reduce your body fat, then opting for main meals that are filling while supporting a calorie deficit, together with some well-planned, measured snacks that keep you within your calorie deficit, is essential.

The problem with snacks is that, sometimes, we don't appreciate the correlation between the volume of food and the caloric value of that food. For example:

- 1 small blueberry muffin (115g)
  = around 5–8 bites of food and 420 calories

- 75g fruit-and-nut mix
  = a handful of food and 360 calories

- 200g fresh strawberries
  = around 15 bites of food and only 60 calories

Choose your snacks wisely and enjoy them.

'BEING GOOD'

30g pistachio nuts	½ medium avocado on a 40g slice of toast
175 cal	265 cal
rice cake & 25g peanut butter	25g mixed seeds
155 cal	143 cal
50g popcorn	40g dark chocolate
244 cal	237 cal

1,219 cal

'BEING BAD'

30g fav choc snack	15g strawberry jam on a 40g slice of toast
152 cal	123 cal
crumpet & 5g butter	25g jelly sweets

140 cal	85 cal
50g tortilla chips	40g milk chocolate
246 cal	214 cal

960 cal

The key to taking control of your dietary outcomes is to understand that there is no good or bad, only different. Understanding nutritional difference enables you to find a balance that supports all aspects of your diet. We know that micronutrients and caloric management are important – but so, too, is enjoyment for long-term adherence. Addressing all these dietary needs by choosing to eat a non-rigid variety of food is the way to achieve all these goals and to realize that 'good' and 'bad' are meaningless terms.

BISCUITS

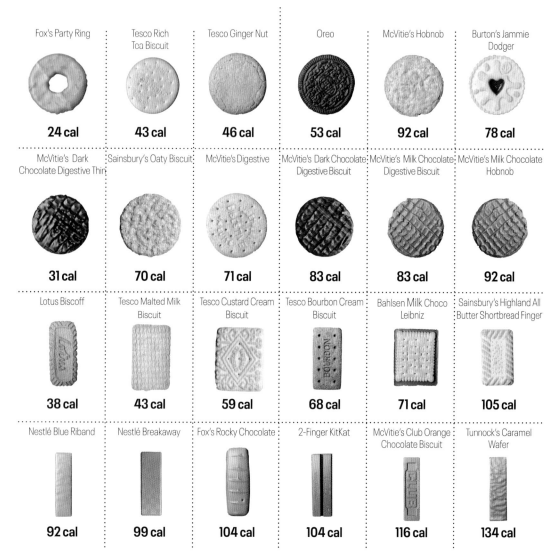

Fox's Party Ring	Tesco Rich Tea Biscuit	Tesco Ginger Nut	Oreo	McVitie's Hobnob	Burton's Jammie Dodger
24 cal	**43 cal**	**46 cal**	**53 cal**	**92 cal**	**78 cal**
McVitie's Dark Chocolate Digestive Thin	Sainsbury's Oaty Biscuit	McVitie's Digestive	McVitie's Dark Chocolate Digestive Biscuit	McVitie's Milk Chocolate Digestive Biscuit	McVitie's Milk Chocolate Hobnob
31 cal	**70 cal**	**71 cal**	**83 cal**	**83 cal**	**92 cal**
Lotus Biscoff	Tesco Malted Milk Biscuit	Tesco Custard Cream Biscuit	Tesco Bourbon Cream Biscuit	Bahlsen Milk Choco Leibniz	Sainsbury's Highland All Butter Shortbread Finger
38 cal	**43 cal**	**59 cal**	**68 cal**	**71 cal**	**105 cal**
Nestlé Blue Riband	Nestlé Breakaway	Fox's Rocky Chocolate	2-Finger KitKat	McVitie's Club Orange Chocolate Biscuit	Tunnock's Caramel Wafer
92 cal	**99 cal**	**104 cal**	**104 cal**	**116 cal**	**134 cal**

There are many more nutritious snacking options than this assortment shows. But there's a reason you've heard of all (or at least most) of them – they are the brands that people enjoy eating the most. And enjoyment should not be underrated. So, instead of assuming biscuits are bad, get to know their place. Enjoy them but make sure you eat micronutrients and a balance of fats, carbs and protein in your overall diet.

'JUST A BISCUIT' AT WORK

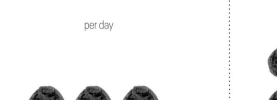

per day

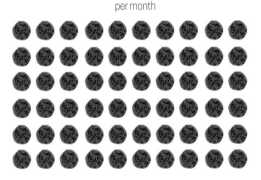

255 cal

per week

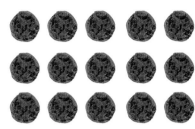

1,275 cal

per month

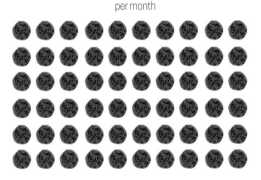

5,100 cal

equivalent to

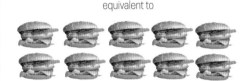

10 Big Macs or...

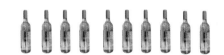

10 x 75cl bottles of white wine

Despite enjoying that biscuit, if you ate three biscuits every day at work over the course of a month, you would be eating the equivalent calories of the McDonald's Big Macs or the bottles of wine displayed here.

Including all the foods you like to eat in your diet is essential to long-term weight-loss success. But, it's vital to realize that some of your favourite snacks add up, over time, to many calories. You might need to adjust other parts of your diet to allow you to include your favourite calorie-dense foods, otherwise they may prevent you from reaching your weight-loss goals.

DOUGHNUTS

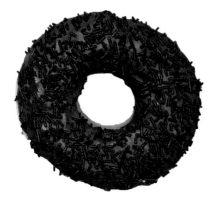
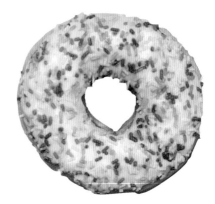

If you love doughnuts, eat them. If you go on a diet that denies you what you love, it will not work.

The realization discussed on the previous page applies to any food, but doughnuts tend to be a common, easy-to-grab and quick-to-eat snack that rapidly accumulates calories.

While munching on a doughnut, know what its calorie implications are and how it fits with your daily and weekly calorie targets.

Eating two doughnuts one day adds around 496 calories. That is a large chunk of your daily energy intake – and they might not fill you up. Basing your snacks on more filling foods while enjoying fewer snacks for fun, in moderation, is a good idea.

You may decide that your overall calorie intake can include that afternoon doughnut, or you may feel that you want to cut down on the number you eat over time. Or perhaps you want to stop eating doughnuts entirely because there is something else that you enjoy even more which contains fewer calories and therefore helps you lose weight.

WHY BREAD DOES NOT MAKE YOU FAT

40g white bread

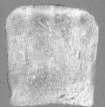

95 cal

40g brown bread

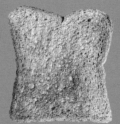

95 cal

+ 30g peanut butter & 20g jam

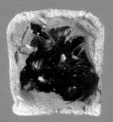

330 cal

+ 30g peanut butter & 20g jam

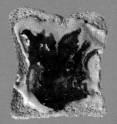

330 cal

When people are trying to lose weight, they think they need to cut out bread from their diet or, at least, replace white bread with wholemeal and brown bread. But, in terms of calories, there is no difference between eating white or brown bread.

It's what you put on top of the bread that you need to keep an eye on. Smearing a couple of generous dollops of peanut butter and jam more than triples the total calorie content of the food you are about to consume.

Don't make bread your enemy. Enjoy bread but consider what you put on top of it. Adding too many calories, not eating bread itself, results in weight gain.

IDOLIZED

DEMONIZED

120g avocado on a 40g slice of brown toast

20g choc & hazelnut spread on a 40g slice of white toast

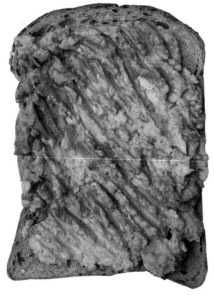

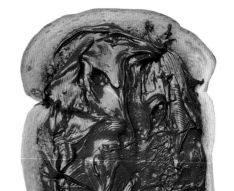

340 cal

203 cal

We idolize some foods because we believe them to be 'better' for us. Similarly, we demonize others that we believe are 'worse' for us. In reality, no food is good or bad when viewed in isolation.

Avocado on brown bread and Nutella on white bread are both are delicious snack options.

In fact, while the avocado toast provides more micronutrients and fibre, it also contains more calories than the portion of Nutella on white bread. Avocado on brown bread is great if you want to increase your micronutrient intake and to feel full for longer, but Nutella toast is a good option if you have already worked micronutrients, protein and fibre into your diet and you want a tasty snack that fits your calorie target. You can also alter the amounts of avocado or Nutella to fit your calorie target.

CHEESE ON TOAST: PORTION CONTROL

TASTY

60g slice sourdough

90g Cheddar cheese

9 small pepperoni slices (30g)

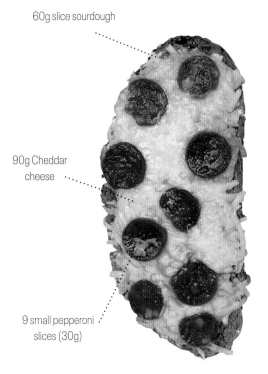

665 cal

STILL TASTY

60g slice sourdough

30g Cheddar cheese

4 pepperoni slices (15g)

2 sliced cherry tomatoes

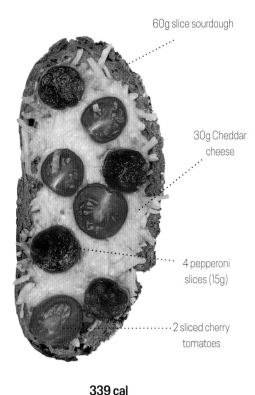

339 cal

Don't try to make drastic changes to your diet overnight. Start by becoming aware and altering the quantities of foods you already consume. This will help you to gradually support your calorie deficit in a familiar and enjoyable way.

You can still eat any food you like, but if fat loss is your goal, then portion control is the way to achieve your calorie target.

This is not rocket science. But it is science.

MORE TOAST IDEAS

5g butter

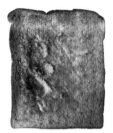

130 cal

¼ medium avocado

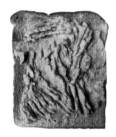

178 cal

20g peanut butter

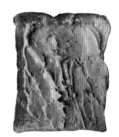

210 cal

1 medium poached egg

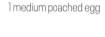
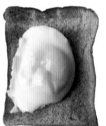

155 cal

¼ medium avocado + 1 medium poached egg

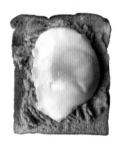

243 cal

20g peanut butter + 5 crushed raspberries

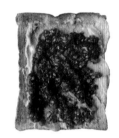

215 cal

2 grilled bacon medallions + 10g ketchup

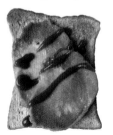

145 cal

20g low-fat Cheddar + 1 slice bresaola, grilled until the cheese is melted

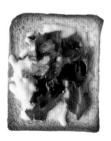

175 cal

¼ medium avocado, 2 grilled bacon medallions + 1 medium poached egg

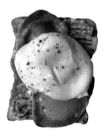

288 cal

CRAVING
CHOCOLATE

Unfulfilling protein cocoa ball thing: 'anything with protein is better than chocolate, right?...'
180 cal

Unfulfilling superfood ball thing: 'check me eating healthily... Who needs chocolate anyway?...'
240 cal

Unfulfilling organic treat thing: 'OK, I miss chocolate. But this is another healthy chocolate-tasting, non-chocolate thing – so it's OK to eat this too...'
150 cal

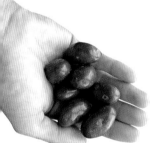

Unfulfilling 85g choc Brazils: 'Getting my healthy fats in like a boss. FYI – still not chocolate so it's cool...'
480 cal

1,050 cal
* didn't really eat chocolate

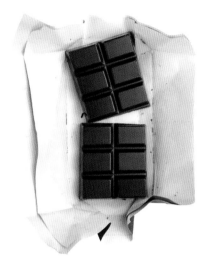

Fulfilling 40g of chocolate: 'because this is what I actually wanted'.

210 cal
* literally ate chocolate

The message here is simple: if you want chocolate, eat it. But if you want to lose fat, be aware of the calorie value of that chocolate.

'Healthier' alternatives often end up being the same or higher in calories than regular chocolate. You can source your micronutrients from your main meals to allow you to enjoy your chocolate!

LOWER-CALORIE SWAPS
THAT TASTE SIMILAR

45g Dairy Milk

240 cal

50g Cheddar

210 cal

18g Freddo

95 cal

50g low-fat Cheddar

145 cal

250g Greek yogurt

233 cal

300ml whole milk

198 cal

250g 0% fat Greek yogurt

135 cal

300ml semi-skimmed milk

150 cal

200ml B&J's choc fudge brownie

418 cal

1,299 cal

200ml Halo Top birthday cake

136 cal

661 cal

The group on the left contains around twice the calories of that on right, yet quantities of both groups are the same (apart from the chocolate). Crucially, the palatable appeal of the lower calorie options is very similar to that of their higher calorie counterparts.

If you recognize opportunities to make small changes that reap handsome long-term rewards, it seems short-sighted not to take them.

PROTEIN-DENSE CONVENIENT SNACKS

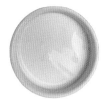

500ml semi-skimmed milk

250 cal

18g protein

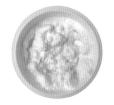

200g fat-free cottage cheese

124 cal

20g protein

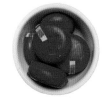

6 Babybel light cheeses

252 cal

30g protein

60g Grenade Caramel Chaos

214 cal

23g protein

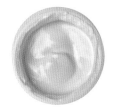

200g 0% fat Greek yogurt

108 cal

21g protein

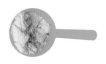

30g flavoured whey powder + water

100 cal

22g protein

100g beef jerky

315 cal

38g protein

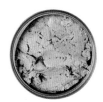

150g canned tuna

170 cal

41g protein

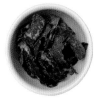

100g beef biltong

278 cal

54g protein

NUTRIENT-DENSE SNACK IDEAS

Here are some easy-to-make snacks to top up your fibre and micronutrient intake between meals.

Smoked salmon on toast

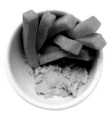

Top a 40g **slice of bread** with 75g of **smoked salmon**.

251 cal

Vanilla & berry protein frozen yogurt

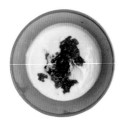

Mix 150g of **0% fat Greek yogurt** with 30g of **vanilla whey protein** powder, 5 **blackberries** and 5 **raspberries**.

198 cal

Chocolate, coconut & strawberry yogurt

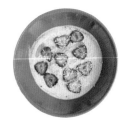

Mix 150g of **0% fat Greek yogurt**, 1 teaspoon **cocoa powder**, 10g **desiccated coconut**, 5g **honey** and 3 chopped **strawberries**.

230 cal

Carrot sticks & guacamole

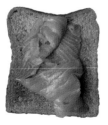

Mash ½ **medium avocado**, the juice from ½ **lime** and ½ teaspoon of **garlic powder** to make guacamole. Chop ½ **medium carrot** into sticks.

190 cal

Almond butter & berry rice cake

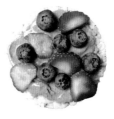

Top a **rice cake** with 30g of **almond butter**, 15g of **blueberries** and 30g of **strawberries**.

240 cal

Peanut butter on sweet potato toast

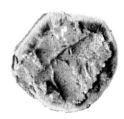

Cut a 50g/1cm-thick slice of **sweet potato**. Toast it in the toaster for 6–8 minutes then add 30g of **peanut butter**.

225 cal

FAST
SNACK IDEAS

When you are really short of time, here are a few super-quick ideas for snacks.

Mozzarella & tomato rice cake

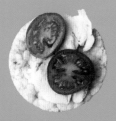

Top a **rice cake** with 50g of fresh **mozzarella** and 1 **cherry tomato**.
155 cal

Garlic avocado mash with chips

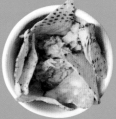

Mash ½ **medium avocado** with 1 teaspoon of **garlic powder** and serve with 6–8 **tortilla chips**.
235 cal

Berry yogurt

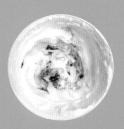

Mix 200g of **0% fat Greek yogurt** with 10 crushed **blackberries** and a drop of **vanilla extract**.
118 cal

Twix

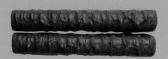

248 cal

BUT I ONLY SNACK ON FRUIT...

(per 100g)

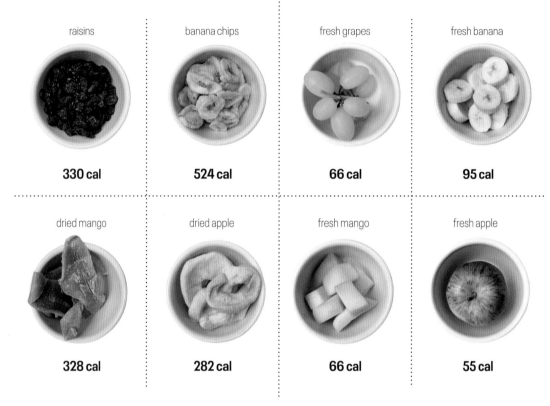

raisins	banana chips	fresh grapes	fresh banana
330 cal	524 cal	66 cal	95 cal

dried mango	dried apple	fresh mango	fresh apple
328 cal	282 cal	66 cal	55 cal

Why are banana chips much higher in calories than fresh bananas? It's a very simple answer. Water makes up 70 per cent of the weight of fresh banana, whereas dried banana loses about 95 per cent of its water content, making it a far more concentrated calorie source. Essentially, per 100g, you're eating the calorie equivalent of five fresh bananas. (Banana chips are dehydrated bananas, which are then coated in oil and sugar, adding more calories than just the fruit.)

This concentration of calories applies to all dried fruit. Diligence is required at all times, even with foods deemed to be 'healthy'.

If fat loss is your goal, it's advisable that you eat fresh fruits instead of dried ones.

FRUIT FACTS

(per 100g)

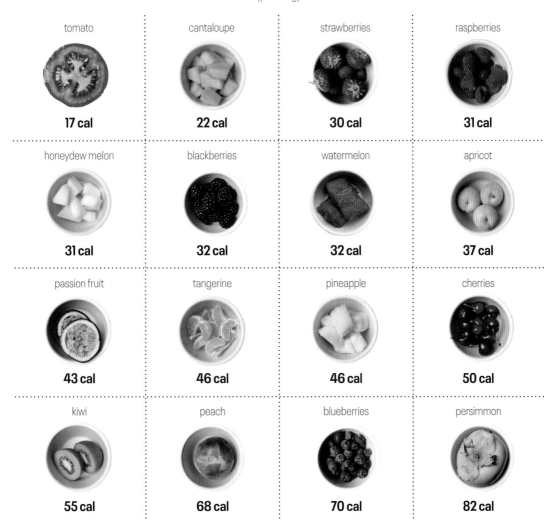

tomato	cantaloupe	strawberries	raspberries
17 cal	**22 cal**	**30 cal**	**31 cal**
honeydew melon	blackberries	watermelon	apricot
31 cal	**32 cal**	**32 cal**	**37 cal**
passion fruit	tangerine	pineapple	cherries
43 cal	**46 cal**	**46 cal**	**50 cal**
kiwi	peach	blueberries	persimmon
55 cal	**68 cal**	**70 cal**	**82 cal**

Despite the cringeworthy term 'nature's candy', most fruit is sweet-tasting and offers vitamins, minerals, fibre and hydrating water, all of which are great for our health. The calories in fruit primarily come from carbohydrates, which is less satisfying than protein, but the fibre content of fruit helps to make you feel full. Fresh fruit, gram per gram, has fewer calories than confectionery. But it still needs to be consumed within your calorie target if you want to lose weight.

READ THE WRAPPER

KitKat Chunky

Eat Natural almond & apricot yogurt bar

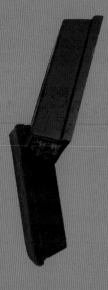

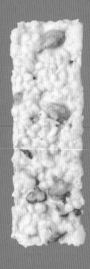

207 cal

247 cal

It is better to read the label to find out if a snack bar fits your energy needs, rather than base your choice on branding alone. For example, this Eat Natural bar has 40 calories more than a KitKat Chunky. The ingredients in the fruit and nut bar are more nutritious, but nutrients will not help with fat loss if the calorie content takes you over your target. Look beyond the brand name and you'll find the key information you need.

'IF I OPEN THE PACKET I'LL EAT THE LOT'

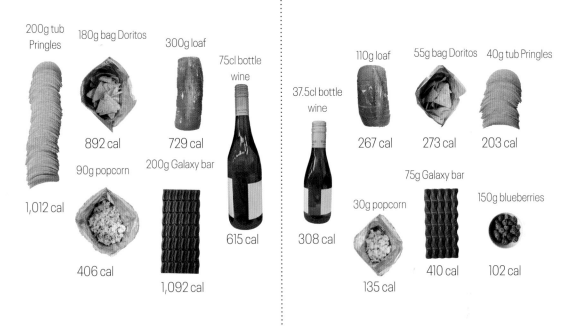

200g tub Pringles
1,012 cal

180g bag Doritos
892 cal

300g loaf
729 cal

75cl bottle wine
615 cal

90g popcorn
406 cal

200g Galaxy bar
1,092 cal

4,746 cal

37.5cl bottle wine
308 cal

110g loaf
267 cal

55g bag Doritos
273 cal

40g tub Pringles
203 cal

30g popcorn
135 cal

75g Galaxy bar
410 cal

150g blueberries
102 cal

1,698 cal

The old saying 'if it's in your cupboard you'll eat it' is true. Why? Because you enjoy that food. But acquiring large packets of calorie-dense snacks can pose a problem, in that we can eat the whole packet once opened instead of the portion that we planned. This is nothing to be ashamed of. However, given the caloric value of some snacks, regularly eating – or drinking – the lot rapidly uses up your overall calorie target for fat loss. A simple solution is to buy a smaller size of the same food. This way you can still consume the whole packet but fewer calories. Win–win. And look to include lower calorie, high-volume foods, too.

CHOOSING
DRINKS

The purpose of drinking liquids is to hydrate and, often, to enjoy the taste. But we need to realize that, just like food, most drinks contain calories.

In some cases, drinks branded with health-based slogans because they contain nutrient-dense ingredients (fresh fruit, for example) can still be relatively high in calories. It is always wise to ignore the marketing promises on the label and judge a drink's merit on its ingredients and nutritional values and how they fit with your weight-loss goal.

It is also worth appreciating the caloric worth of the likes of coffee and alcoholic drinks so that you can make adjustments to your diet to include drinks you really enjoy.

The realization that there are lower-calorie alternatives to your favourite drinks also offers a great opportunity to experience a similar taste while supporting your weight-loss goal.

One source of hydration that contains zero calories is water. To stay hydrated we should drink at least 2 litres of water every day. Staying hydrated is essential for our organs to function, from absorbing nutrients from our food and aiding digestion to keeping our brains alert and our skin supple. Contrary to water being 'boring' and tasteless, flavoured/sparkling versions are available that also amount to zero calories.

BEING HEALTHY

BEING RIDICULOUS

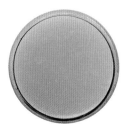

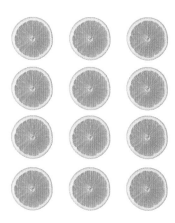

500ml orange juice
(6 small oranges)

6 small oranges

190 cal

190 cal

The idea of drinking 500ml of orange juice to quench your thirst seems legitimate – and it is, if you enjoy it – whereas the thought of consuming six small oranges in one sitting seems ridiculous. Yet the irony is that either option provides exactly the same caloric values. Just because you're not eating food doesn't mean that the calories do not exist – you need to factor in the calories in drinks, too.

An orange juice might seem a healthy choice, but since one glass or bottle contains the equivalent calories and sugar, as well as micronutrients, as six whole oranges, does drinking the juice help or hinder you achieving your calorie target?

Lately, there's been a craze for homemade juices and smoothies. While these are a source of nutrients, don't forget that homemade drinks still count towards your daily calorie intake and, depending on ingredients, can be caloric. In fact, eating fruit and vegetables is a better option than drinking juices/smoothies because you consume the fibre they contain, which is important for feeling full and better digestion.

JUST A COFFEE

(per week)

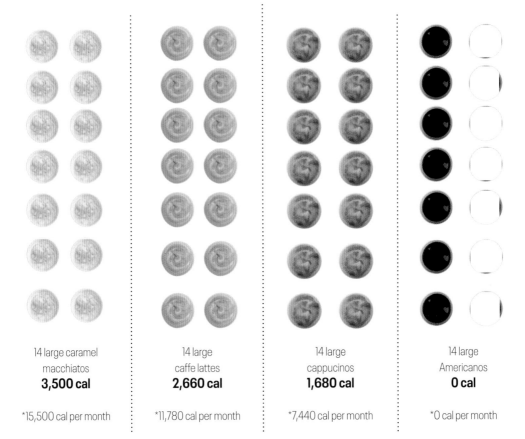

14 large caramel macchiatos	14 large caffe lattes	14 large cappucinos	14 large Americanos
3,500 cal	**2,660 cal**	**1,680 cal**	**0 cal**
*15,500 cal per month	*11,780 cal per month	*7,440 cal per month	*0 cal per month

Black coffee (with no added milk, sugar or flavourings) contains virtually zero calories and therefore does not need to enter the calorie-counting equation. Although we refer to all coffee drinks as 'coffee', lattes, mochas and other flavoured coffees pose different caloric propositions.

If you are drinking multiple cups of these drinks every day in a bid to 'perk up', you need to consider the total calories consumed and how this affects your calorie requirements for the day and week.

It is also worth considering your choice of milk (see page 98) and the size of the drinks you consume – the larger the drink, the greater its caloric value.

TEA/COFFEE SWAPS

Tea	Tea + 10 ml semi-skimmed milk	Tea + 10ml semi-skimmed milk + 1 tsp sugar	Green tea	Fruit tea
0 cal	5 cal	37 cal	0 cal	5 cal

medium Americano	medium latte*	medium caramel latte*	medium cappuccino*	medium mocha*
0 cal	103 cal	257 cal	90 cal	237 cal

large Americano	large latte*	large caramel latte*	large cappuccino*	large mocha*
0 cal	141 cal	346 cal	119 cal	353 cal

* all based on skimmed milk

If you like to drink tea or coffee, consider the calories and make sure it is not taking you over your calorie target. Can you switch your tea/coffee preference – make it smaller and choose less milk?

SMOOTHIE

COLA

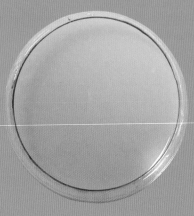

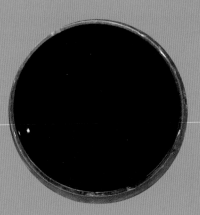

750ml smoothie

750ml cola

432 cal

315 cal

Despite smoothies and juices containing fruit or vegetables, some are calorie dense.

That is because a large amount of fruit is puréed into the product – in the case of the one above: 4 pressed apples, 1 mashed banana, 20 white grapes, ½ crushed mango and ½ crushed kiwi. Cola is low in nutrients. But calories, not nutrients, determine body fat. So cola could be a more useful choice for weight loss than this smoothie, if it fits within your calorie target!

'MAKES YOU SLIM'
(per week)

3 × 360ml green smoothies
+ 4 × red smoothies

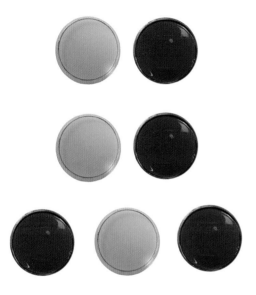

1,350 cal

'MAKES YOU FAT'
(per week)

3 x fizzy orange, 2 x lemonade, 2 x reduced sugar cola

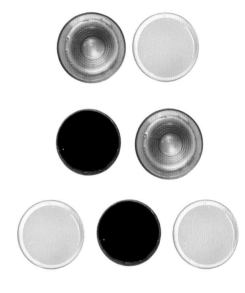

411 cal

*Don't confuse nutrient intake with energy balance

Over time, despite the intake of micronutrients, calories consumed from smoothies and juices can add up. If you enjoy them, then drink them. But remember to factor them into your overall daily and weekly calorie targets.

OKAY, BETTER, BEST ...

OKAY...

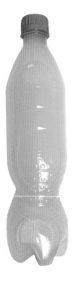

500ml UK Fanta
95 cal

if you enjoy the drink and are aware of the calories/sugar density within your overall diet so that moderate consumption still supports your nutritional goals.

BETTER...

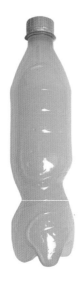

500ml UK Fanta Zero
19 cal

if you regularly consume the full-calorie version and want to aid a calorie deficit by consuming virtually no calories or sugar from a drink that you enjoy.

BEST...

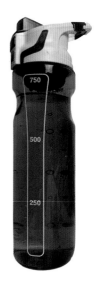

0 cal

if you want to stay hydrated, consume zero calories/sugar/non-optimal ingredients, and help the environment by cutting down on single-use plastic.

Fizzy drinks are often blamed for contributing to obesity. This is mainly due to their lack of fibre, meaning that you are very unlikely to feel full after drinking them and therefore more likely to consume greater quantities, hence more calories. The bottom line is: it's okay to drink calorie-dense drinks if you enjoy them and appreciate their caloric worth. It's better to source lower-calorie versions of your favourite drink, if fat loss is the aim, and you drink them a lot. But it's best to get your hydration from water – and especially if you fill a reusable bottle to help the environment by reducing your single-use plastic consumption.

PROTEIN SHAKE

PROTEIN MEAL

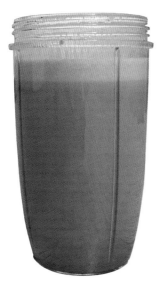

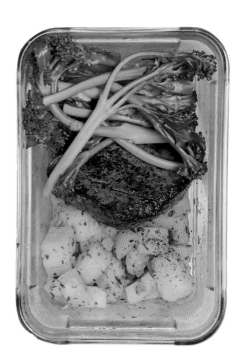

protein consumed

protein still consumed
* additional nutritional benefits

Protein shakes are superb sources of convenient protein, if you're short on time or on the go. However, as long as you consume sufficient protein throughout the day, you can maintain muscle without recourse to protein shakes.

The protein in many protein shakes is whey, an excellent, cost-effective source of dense protein. But this is no better than the protein you can obtain from eating meat, fish, eggs or milk. Eating a meal containing the same amount of protein as a shake does the same job while providing additional nutrients. Contrary to claims, protein shakes do not have magical powers to help you lose weight.

WHAT HAPPENS WHEN YOU DRINK DIET/ZERO-CALORIE FIZZY DRINK

'I'll get cancer because diet coke contains aspartame.'.

'It tricks my brain into releasing insulin, which will give me type II diabetes.'

'One can of diet coke will destroy my gut health and lead to disease.'

'I've heard you can clean silver with diet coke, so it must be bad.'

'Drinking diet coke will make me fat, unlike smoothies or juices.'

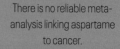

There is no reliable meta-analysis linking aspartame to cancer.

Diet coke contains no calories and no sugar, therefore there is no insulin response.

Excessive consumption may negatively impact on your gut microbiome. But moderate consumption will not.

A silver coin does not replicate the human anatomy.

Diet coke has zero calories and contains no sugar, unlike smoothies or juices.

The assumption that diet drinks are 'bad' has been borne out of the nutrition industry's innate ability to ignore science and spread pseudoscientific pandemonium.

The concern that 'aspartame causes cancer and other diseases' has not been proven by any reputable studies. One study conducted on rats suggests a possible link to blood cancers, but we are not rats. The largest study conducted on 500,000 humans found no link between aspartame and any form of cancer.

The belief that 'sweeteners trick our brains into thinking we've eaten sugar, causing an insulin response' also flounders because there are no calories or sugar in diet drinks. No insulin response is possible.

Many newspapers have printed that 'diet drinks cause obesity,' but have been unable to source reliable information to back up such a claim. It is not possible to gain fat if zero calories are consumed.

The truth is that diet drinks are neither good nor bad and you can drink them as part of a nutrient-dense, energy-controlled diet.

NIGHT OUT

An evening out would be fairly dull if it didn't involve a degree of indulgence, be that food or alcohol. One night out a month won't make a big impact on fat loss; regular nights out every week will.

For example, if your calorie target for fat loss is 1,800 calories per day or 12,600 calories per week (this varies from person to person), the items consumed in the left column equate to two-thirds of your total weekly calorie allowance, but are consumed in just 36 hours. Even by 'getting back on track' the following day, and eating 1,800 calories, your weekly calorie target is busted.

Instead of wondering why you can't lose fat because you're 'on track' most of the time, recognize where you are going wrong. You can make better choices on your nights out and reduce their regularity. Nights out should not be spent worrying about the nutritional values of food/drinks, but if you're well informed, you can stay within your calorie target and still have fun.

STAGE 1
Dinner

starter
300 cal

pizza
1,200 cal

2 x 250ml
white wine
350 cal

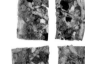

garlic bread
350 cal

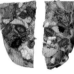

STAGE 1
Dinner

starter
300 cal

pizza
1,200 cal

1 x 250ml
white wine
175 cal

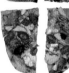

STAGE 2
Go to a bar and club and drink like a fish

1 x 250ml
white wine
175 cal

2 x
double g&t
360 cal

3 x
Jägerbombs
630 cal

2 x
tequilas
130 cal

STAGE 2
Go to a bar and club and enjoy yourself

4 x
gin and slimline
tonics 240 cal

1 x
Jägerbomb
210 cal

1 x
tequila
65 cal

and be in a fit
state to talk to
people

STAGE 3
get a kebab and try not to
drop it down your front

Doner kebab & chips
1,400 cal

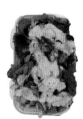

THE NEXT DAY
bedridden malaise followed
by these:

burritos, large fries, 3 cookies,
packet of M&Ms + tub of B&J's
4,310 cal

9,205 cal

STAGE 3
go to bed
(yours or someone else's)

sleep/fun
0 cal/300 cal

THE NEXT DAY
more hanky panky and return
to nutritional norm

1 cookie, 100g raspberries,
250g yogurt/berries,
2 x 600 cal meals
1,800 cal

3,990 cal

ALCOHOLIC DRINKS, SPIRITS & MIXERS

With drinks that tend to be consumed 'straight', such as lager, beer or wine, it's the alcohol volume (%ABV on the label) that determines some of the calorie content. So choosing a beverage with a lower ABV will result in fewer calories being consumed from alcohol. But bear in mind that calories are often added to beers, ciders and wines in the form of carbohydrates. In spirits, the ABV is higher, but the measure is usually much smaller – here it's the mixers that can load on the calories, again usually in the form of carbohydrates.

250ml vodka diet coke

60 cal

40ml tequila shot

65 cal

125ml champagne flute

90 cal

125ml glass of prosecco

93 cal

250ml measure Southern Comfort & lemonade

95 cal

40ml whisky

97 cal

250ml martini

103 cal

250ml can of vodka cranberry

110 cal

250ml single gin & tonic

110 cal

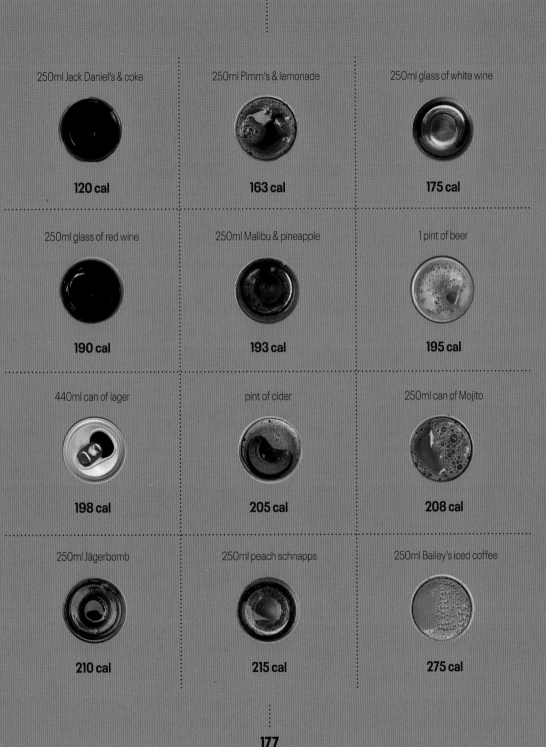

250ml Jack Daniel's & coke

120 cal

250ml Pimm's & lemonade

163 cal

250ml glass of white wine

175 cal

250ml glass of red wine

190 cal

250ml Malibu & pineapple

193 cal

1 pint of beer

195 cal

440ml can of lager

198 cal

pint of cider

205 cal

250ml can of Mojito

208 cal

250ml Jägerbomb

210 cal

250ml peach schnapps

215 cal

250ml Bailey's iced coffee

275 cal

HOW TO
EXERCISE

When we exercise we use energy. If our goal is to reduce body fat, exercising regularly is a good idea as it increases the number of calories that we burn. What many of us don't realize, however, is that we burn calories just by existing. Exercise offers a short, intense opportunity to burn calories, but it's not the only way to lose weight. Quite often, when we start a weight-loss regime, we set unrealistic targets of exercising every day that very quickly fall away because they are unsustainable.

If you're very active you will require more calories to achieve a sustainable calorie deficit. If you are sedentary, sitting at a desk most of the day, you will require fewer calories to achieve a sustainable calorie deficit.

I have been asked thousands of times what the best fat-loss exercise is. My answer remains the same: none.

There is no single mode of exercise that helps fat loss more than another. Energy is not only burned by HIIT (high-intensity interval training), expensive DVDs and CrossFit classes. In fact, although you would still be using energy, strenuous activity will likely only account for 5–10 per cent of your total daily energy expenditure because you cannot do intense exercise for long periods. The type of exercise that will help you lose fat is the one you enjoy and can fit into your life regularly.

If you don't enjoy the exercise you're doing, you won't keep it up for long. Whether you embark on HIIT, CrossFit, exercise classes, powerlifting, bodybuilding, Pilates, running marathons, walking or your own exercise programme, do it because you enjoy it, not because it's a means to an end or because it looks cool on Instagram.

CARDIO OR WEIGHTS?

Put simply, neither one is better than the other for fat loss.

It's a common misconception that cardio is more beneficial than weights for fat loss because being out of breath, increasing your heart rate or sweating are all signs of strenuous physical activity. But breathing heavily is merely the body's way of trying to take in more oxygen, an increased heart rate reflects the need to pump more blood to circulate that oxygen around the body, and sweating is the body's way of cooling down – none of which directly results in more fat loss.

Resistance training (weight training) often results in fewer immediate signs of strain, but that doesn't mean that the same – or more – energy is not being used. Energy is required to lift heavy weights, but the symptom of exertion here is muscular fatigue. Research has shown that our resting metabolism is elevated for longer after weight training than after cardio.

Weight training can be great for goal-based improvements, motivating you to progress to lifting heavier weights or managing more reps to build strength as well as burn fat.

HIIT (high-intensity interval training) has risen to fame in the past few years but it is not magical. In fact, the impact on joints from jumping around can put them under unnecessary pressure. HIIT requires only a small amount of time, which makes it an attractive option, although it still has to be enjoyable or you simply won't do it regularly.

The bottom line is: do the exercise that suits you and that you enjoy the most. Whichever you choose, the key for fat loss is the frequency of the exercise and the calories burned while doing it, not the type of exercise.

YOU DON'T NEED TO JOIN A GYM

You don't need to take out a gym membership to lose weight. If you find public gyms intimidating or they make you feel uncomfortable, you don't need to go there. Many people join gyms in January with a commitment to visit five times per week, then barely turn up all year. After the excesses of the festive period, and subsequent New Year resolve to shed the pounds, most people realize they don't know what to do in a gym or that they don't have enough time to commute to and from the gym, and quickly give up.

It's better to set realistic goals that can be achieved inside or outside a gym. Calorie intake should be calculated according to the amount of exercise and day-to-day movement you do. For example, a 75kg (11.8-stone) female who exercises five times per week will need to consume more calories than a 75kg female who exercises once or twice per week in order for the calorie deficit to be sustainable for gradual fat loss.

Outside the gym environment, there are many easy opportunities to burn energy and lose fat that do not involve planned exercise. Read on to find out more.

HOW WE BURN ENERGY

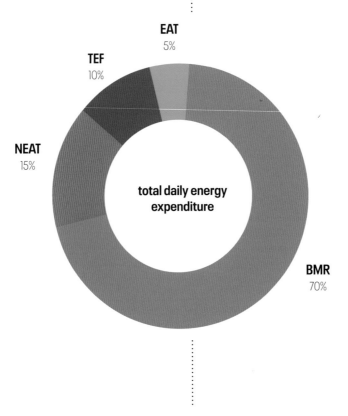

EAT
5%

TEF
10%

NEAT
15%

total daily energy
expenditure

BMR
70%

Even if you do no exercise, you burn energy every day. Total daily energy expenditure is comprised of: **BMR** (basal metabolic rate) – energy burned when at rest, just by existing; **TEF** (thermic effect of food) – energy burned during the metabolization of food; **EAT** (exercise activity thermogenesis) – energy burned during planned exercise; and **NEAT** (non-exercise activity thermogenesis) – energy burned during all unplanned movement, often when performing day-to-day tasks such as walking, ironing or fidgeting.

NINE WAYS TO INCREASE YOUR NEAT

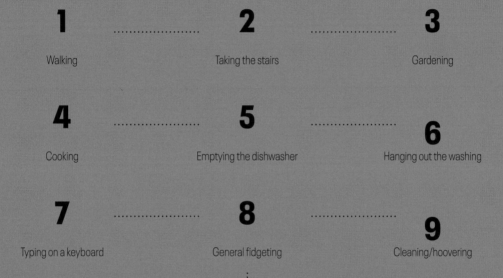

1 Walking

2 Taking the stairs

3 Gardening

4 Cooking

5 Emptying the dishwasher

6 Hanging out the washing

7 Typing on a keyboard

8 General fidgeting

9 Cleaning/hoovering

The significance of taking a daily ten-minute walk seems small, but over time those ten minutes of movement amount to extra energy expenditure, creating a greater calorie deficit and quicker fat loss. Consider all of these ways to increase your NEAT as the aspect of your weight-loss journey that you can easily chip away at every day with minimal planning or upheaval.

WHY 'NEAT' IS KEY FOR FAT LOSS

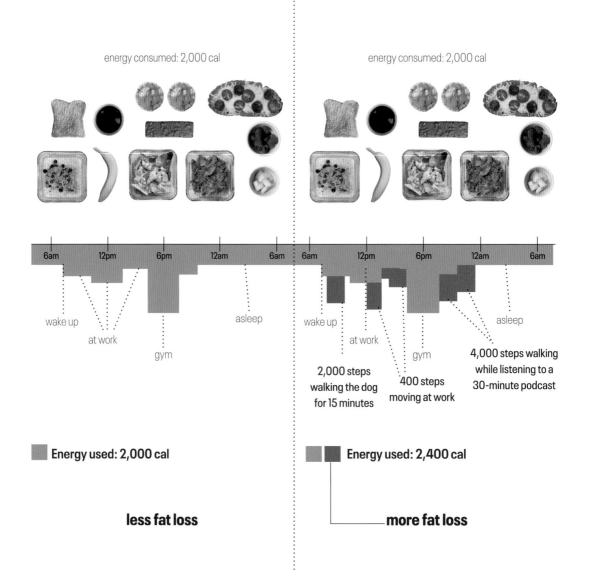

energy consumed: 2,000 cal

energy consumed: 2,000 cal

6am 12pm 6pm 12am 6am

6am 12pm 6pm 12am 6am

wake up

at work

gym

asleep

wake up

at work

gym

asleep

2,000 steps
walking the dog
for 15 minutes

400 steps
moving at work

4,000 steps walking
while listening to a
30-minute podcast

Energy used: 2,000 cal

Energy used: 2,400 cal

less fat loss

more fat loss

While you are urged to 'hit the gym', reminded of your exercise shortcomings and told that you 'just don't want it enough', there lurks something stupendously simple that could provide a formidable opportunity for fat-loss progress – **NEAT**.

The graphic here shows two identical dietary intakes of 2,000 calories (yours will be individual to you). But, crucially, due to the increase in NEAT in the example on the right, the energy expenditure is higher than in the example on the left. NEAT is the variable that creates this greater energy deficit, resulting in a greater reduction in body fat.

Despite planned exercise being advantageous too, the beauty of NEAT is that you do not need to take out a gym membership, learn perfect technique, pay a PT £50 an hour or do burpees. Instead, you simply need to move more, and more often.

Achieving maximum rewards with minimal upheaval will make it easier to make sustainable lifestyle changes. Increasing NEAT to reduce body fat goes against everything the industry tells you to do, but its simplicity may be one of the catalysts to your success.

As NEAT plays an important role in your energy expenditure (and, therefore, calorie deficit) over time, make sure your deficit is not too aggressive (see pages 38–9). Often the temptation is to seek rapid weight loss, but if you consume too few calories you won't have the energy for NEAT. Organizing a gradual calorie deficit which gives you enough energy to move more and not feel exhausted or hungry is best for successful long-term weight loss.

THE FASTED EXERCISE MYTH

FASTED EXERCISE

(Train on an empty stomach)

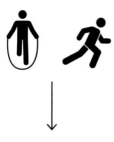

then eat breakfast

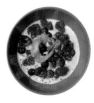

560 calories consumed after energy is used from exercise

FED EXERCISE

(Eat at some point before you exercise)

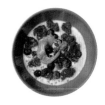

wait a while before exercising...

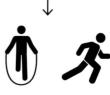

still 560 calories consumed after energy is used from exercise

The key here is to understand the difference between fat oxidation and fat loss. Fat oxidation is the process of fat turning into energy, whereas fat loss is the process of fat mass decreasing. When we eat, we secrete insulin. This results in less fat oxidation, meaning less fat is available to be used as energy. This does not stop fat loss from occurring because, as we know, fat loss is only governed by total energy in versus energy out. Not eating a meal before exercise first thing in the morning means that fat is the only energy source for your body to burn. Many think this will result in more fat loss, but it's actually just more fat oxidation.

Anyone claiming that fasted exercise results in greater fat loss is misunderstanding the science.

WHY YOU DON'T NEED
TO TRACK CALORIES BURNED

fitness tracker

The latest high-tech
fitness tracker

**That run burned
328 calories,
Sally, well done!**

the reality

The latest high-tech
fitness tracker

**It cannot predict
the exact calories
you burn**

Given that it's a very good idea to be aware of calories or track them when trying to lose or gain weight, surely it's also a good idea to track calories burned?

No.

The reason for this is simple: the calories on food labels are accurate; the calories estimated by tracking apps and watches are not. These devices can give you a ballpark figure, but it's impossible for them to tell you how many calories you're actually burning. What you can be sure of is that by regularly moving and exercising you will be using energy, which will help you lose fat. Using these trackers to set progressive goals, such as increasing reps or step targets, and tracking the regularity of your movement rather than the exact number of calories burned, will be much more beneficial to you.

CONCLUSION–
HOW WILL YOU LOSE WEIGHT?

clean eating?

meal replacements?

raw food?

supplements?

slimming club?

diet tea?

paleo?

vegan?

alkaline?

5:2?

YOUR DIET

STAY INSIDE THE CIRCLE
AS NOTHING ON THE OUTSIDE
IS NECESSARY

vegetarian?

detox?

keto?

juicing?

low carb?

cleanse?

organic?

intermittent fasting?

Eat fewer calories and move more
in a way that you can sustain

Life after the calorie deficit

After losing weight, people often gain that weight back over time. This is usually because people don't understand how they lost weight, and how it may be gained again. You now understand exactly how to lose weight in a sustainable way (see pages 38–9). When you reach a point where you no longer want to lose weight, the amount of calories you consume and expend at this point becomes your maintenance balance of energy. You may want to keep tracking calories consumed or you may be skilled enough to eyeball portion sizes after educating yourself with the tools that this book provides.

Now that you have reached the end of this book, hopefully you will have ditched all the misleading, mythical and error-laden ideas about food and weight loss.

Mindset is key to all the decisions we make in life. A mind freed from the clutter of guilt, shame and fear is a mind that is ready to implement its fact-based understanding of food.

- You are armed with the ability to sniff out and avoid bullsh*t claims, fads and diet culture.

- You can cut through popular pseudoscience and complicated dieting rhetoric.

- You have all the knowledge required to lose, or gain, or simply maintain your weight.

- You can take complete control of what and when you eat and drink, and how you exercise.

- You are in a strong place, diet culture cannot touch you.

- You are powerful.

You may have finished reading this book, but let it be a constant source of information, reassurance and companionship on your journey to making empowering changes in your life.

INDEX

ACKNOWLEDGEMENTS

Firstly, I would like to thank you for choosing to spend your money to buy my book. I am truly grateful that you have put your faith in me to help you on your journey. Now it's time to have faith in yourself. You are now empowered with the knowledge you need to eat what you like, enjoy it and lose weight, if you wish.

I owe a tremendous amount of gratitude to my Instagram following around the world who have supported me from the start. Without your faith, this book may never have been published. I've shared just a very small amount of the direct messages I have received on the endpapers of this book. Thank you.

Putting this book together has been a colossal effort from myself and my publishing team. I would like to thank Ebury and Penguin for putting their faith in my idea and providing the launch pad for it to flourish; and Sophie Yamamoto, the book designer, for her careful attention to detail. Thank you for making publishing my first book an enjoyable, relaxed experience.

A special thanks also goes to Jen, my agent, (and the rest of the team) who have always been there throughout, putting their faith in me from day one.

Thank you to my parents for raising me to fight for what is right and to refuse to accept what is wrong.

10 9 8 7 6 5 4 3 2 1

Ebury Press, an imprint of Ebury Publishing,
20 Vauxhall Bridge Road,
London, SW1V 2SA

Ebury Press is part of the Penguin Random House group of companies whose addresses can be found at global.penguinrandomhouse.com

 Penguin Random House UK

Text and Illustrations Copyright © Graeme Tomlinson 2020

Graeme has asserted his right to be identified as the author of this Work in accordance with the Copyright, Designs and Patents Act 1988

Additional photo credits: Bottles on pages 31, 37, 38, 39, 44 and 58 © stockphoto-graf; diet coke can on page 38 and 39 © Africa Studio; coke can on page 38 and 44 © Karandaev; toothpaste tube on page 84 © Maksym Yemelyanov; phone on page 58 © Fenskey; fried chicken on page 65 © Uros Pretovic; fries on page 65 © Idler Akhmerov; red cross on page 88, 92 and 172 © Brovarky; Bed on page 175 © 2dmolier. All Adobe Stock Images.

First published by Ebury Press in 2020

www.penguin.co.uk

A CIP catalogue record for this book is available from the British Library

ISBN: 978 1 529 10604 6

Designed by maru studio
Colour origination by Rhapsody Ltd London
Printed and bound in Italy by L.E.G.O. S.p.A

Penguin Random House is committed to a sustainable future for our business, our readers and our planet. This book is made from Forest Stewardship Council® certified paper.

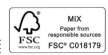

MIX
Paper from responsible sources
FSC® C018179
www.fsc.org

'For 10 years now I have struggled to understand why I can't look a certain way. I am in week 5 of a calorie deficit, and it has been the most eye-opening experience of my life. I am beginning to see results when I put on my clothes and when I look in the mirror, it's incredible. Thank you massively!' Mia, UK

'Lost 40kg this year in a healthy way. Thanks for keeping it real. You've helped me understand food and nutrition. Sending love and respect your way bro.' Muhammad, UK

'Learning about what I put into my body has been super helpful. Thanks for endless inspiration and education.' Michaela, Sweden

'I now know that one 'junk meal' doesn't wreck my day anymore because I look at the week. One 'ruined' meal out of twenty isn't that dire. I know I can eat out and I know how to plan my meals. I can make smart choices today and better choices tomorrow. Thank you for recalibrating my outlook.' Jenifer, USA

'Your posts have taught me to be more confident about my food choices as long as they are balanced. Your account is like an oasis on Instagram. The internet needs more people like you.' Hilary, Hong Kong

'I've had a very unhealthy relationship with food and body image from a young teen and for the last couple of years have been obsessed with following weight-loss accounts and influencers. Since finding your page and disassociating food with being 'bad' I am no longer in a vicious cycle of punishing myself, and I have an appreciation for what my body is capable of.' Rebecca, UK

'I've never felt so much freedom with food and I've lost 30 pounds in over 8 months!' Lisa, UK